WHITE FLAG

Discovering the power of the mind:
A path out of infertility pain

WHITE
FLAG

Shannon Weber

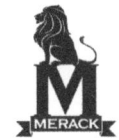

Published and distributed by Merack Publishing
California, USA

Library of Congress Control Number: 2024918256
Weber, Shannon
White Flag
ISBN Paperback: 978-1-957048-41-3
Hardcover: 978-1-957048-42-0
eBook: 978-1-964421-00-1

Contents

Chapter 1

The Making of an Unraveled Woman

"There is a unique pain that comes from preparing a place in your heart for a child that never comes."

DAVID PLATT

I was out of toilet paper. When I stood up from the toilet and reached for another roll, there it was, a drop of blood on the white tile of my bathroom floor. I could almost hear the sound of the drip ricocheting off the ceramic tile. I stared in silence at what the sight of blood signaled to me: the death of a monthly dream. After seventy-two months of routine heartache, my period no longer connected me to fertility and life; it only served as a reminder of my biggest failure in life. I was still not pregnant. The blood denied me the one experience I wanted most: motherhood.

I had never failed at anything in my life before this. Years before, as a fierce thirteen year old, I had an experience that taught me I was built to win. I grew up in a small town of about 17,000 people outside Dallas, Texas. It was a big deal when we got a second grocery store.

But the town survived with just one Dairy Queen and one Stop N Go gas station. Cheering was a big deal at my high school (well, in the whole state of Texas), and I enjoyed being a cheerleader for the Coppell Cowboys—wearing red, white, and black, and yelling on the sidelines for football and basketball games. I was lucky enough to make the squad each year, but the tryouts were by far the scariest thing I had ever done at this stage in life. By the time I was a Senior, trying out in front of the whole school got much easier, but when I was in the eighth grade and thirteen years old, I had to try out by myself on stage in front of the entire high school in the dome auditorium. I literally thought I would die right there in front of all of the "older" high school people, the SENIORS. Wearing red shorts and a white shirt, with my hair in a ponytail tied in a red ribbon, there I was, five-foot-nothing, waiting my turn to walk out on the stage to perform my cheer and do a jump in front of four hundred-plus kids, teachers, and parents.

Oh my God. How am I going to do this?

I was holding my breath without even knowing it. My eyes were wide, and my eyebrows stretched high to the top of my face.

I could see all the people sitting down in the auditorium as I peered past the red velvet curtain. The room was full. I felt fear. Fear of failure. Not knowing what to do. My heart was beating 200 beats per minute. Terror in this moment was an understatement.

What if I freeze up there, or I can't remember the words, or I fall down? Oh my God, they are all going to laugh at me, and then I will not be able to step foot into this high school.

But I signed up for this. This is what I wanted, and there was no backing out now. If I made a run for it, I would definitely be the laughing-stock of the eighth graders. Doomed for all of high school. I finally remembered to breathe and took a deep breath in, and then another as I watched the girl before me walk off the stage. Then I heard my name called. I took one more deep breath and pulled it deep down inside my body, to the deepest part of my belly. It was there that I found my strength, my power waiting for me to connect. As I gently released my breath through my nose, I felt the calm wash over me.

Fuck it. Let's do this.

I walked out on the wooden stage as a plank creaked beneath me. The stage lights were bright, which helped me block out the crowd and tune into my cheer. As I reached my mark and stood before all of my peers, staring back at me in silence, I took a second to take it all in.

Wow. That's a lot of people.

I realized it was not that scary once I stood right in my fear. I actually had found my courage waiting for me, but I had to step into the fear to find it. This lesson will be unlearned and learned again over and over in my infertile adult years. Irony at its finest.

I smiled big as the crowd cheered for me when I walked off the stage. I was loud, I didn't forget my cheer—and I made the squad.

I suppose I have always been super loud to compensate for my short lady syndrome. Yes, I can admit this. I was loud all the time, mostly because I was excited about everything and wanted everyone else to be excited too. Cheering was a natural thing for me to do. Here, I had the perfect outlet to yell and scream in front of people. I was so loud that my friends could hear me from the parking lot!

When I met my husband, I was still loud and proud. Maybe that was the Texan in me, a characteristic well-known to everybody. He loved that about me. In those days we enjoyed snowboarding together. Amid our struggle with infertility, the memory of a particular day spent snowboarding (which turned out to be less than ideal) would frequently resurface in my mind. I wondered, was this memory a message, the reason we were having trouble conceiving?

It was the winter before we were married, and John and I spent most of our time snowboarding. I thought of myself as a really good rider, until the mountain taught me a lesson. A lesson that would come back to me over and over during our infertility journey.

I was confident and liked to go fast. I craved the ease of the glide through fresh powder, but the quiet stillness of the mountain is what I connected with most. There is a certain serenity received from the mountain, and it was felt as we rested between runs and sat against the mountainside, leaning on our knees, scanning the horizon and valley below. Such beauty left us without words. When you can see as far as the sky reaches, this expansiveness of vision radiates your soul. In this place, I am in the moment, fully present, resting in my true peace. In this peace, I feel connected and in tune with my life, in the flow of everything, with no resistance of any kind. Here, I can do anything because life feels easy; it is easy. It's like I can think anything and make it happen, come to life, like fruition is my superpower.

Life was simple and carefree in those days, with little responsibility and children far from my desire. I never imagined I would be one to crash into a tree, but I did. We were riding fast down an easy green when another skier came to a dead stop in my path with no time for me to get out of it. It was either him or the giant pine tree. I remember lying there in shock after the impact. I could not feel the center of my body until I tried to move, and a shot of searing pain exploded through my core. My mind began to process the situation as the panic set in. *Oh shit, oh shit. Is this a Sonny Bono moment? Am I gonna fade to black and be done? Is this it?* Then, I heard a voice calmly say in a John Wayne kind of way, "Not even close." And for a moment, it was as if someone had pushed pause on my life. It was a bluebird day on the mountain, and I could see the sun shining through the tree branches above. The wind whispered softly through the mountain air, and in that stillness, that familiar moment of peace washed over me.

My official prognosis was a broken pelvis in six places and three broken ribs. To my surprise, my first question was, "Am I going to be able to have children?"

The doctor hesitated before leaving the room, almost surprised I had asked the question. He looked back over his shoulder as he said, "You should be fine to bear children."

I laid my head back down on the hospital bed. Even then, I knew he had no fucking idea if that was true.

A year after my accident, on the morning of our wedding, we shared coffee together on the back deck. I could see the blue sky again after days of smoke-filled skies from the forest fires. It had been very hot, low 90s, but not today. For our special day, Montana gave us 78 degrees. We sat in silence and smiled deeply at one another. Like the subtle scents of a lilac flower, our smiles shared the promise of sweetness, filled with our love and respect for one another. This was it, the reason we were doing this. This was our connection. It was easy and simple, and we both believed in it. When it was time to leave the house, knowing the next time we saw each other would be at the altar, he grabbed my face and kissed me deeply. No words were needed. Our green and hazel eyes said it all. *This feels good. This is right, in sickness and in health.*

Before leaving our wedding, I had a nudge to stop, turn around, and take in the scene. I wanted to imprint and capture this memory in time. As I looked out into the ceremony site, the serene feeling of the moment was set by the sway of the white-strung lights throughout the apple trees and around the gazebo draped with flowers that served as our altar. Present in the sky was the waning crescent moon, high above the mountains, surrounded by stars glistening down on us. We created magic here today, our magic, to be carried into a beautiful life together. I stood there in gratitude and soaked in all the goodness of this moment filled with such peace, joy, and happiness. My heart was full, and I wanted to remember what a full heart felt like. I took a deep breath in before leaving this moment and saw the black cat that jumped on my dress during the ceremony sitting on a nearby rock wall. He wagged his tail from side to side and let out a goodbye meow. I sat beside him, gave him a pet, and silently thanked him for blessing our wedding day.

Like all newlyweds, we shared the desire to have a family. Since we married later in life and were in our early thirties now, we started trying to get pregnant right away. We had been trying for one full year before deciding to speak to an infertility doctor, because that's what the internet told us to do. Officially entering the infertility world was inconceivable to me. I was in shock that I had to make an appointment with an infertility specialist, much less go through treatments of any kind. I still had to remind myself to breathe because the weight of the worry was beginning to press down hard on my chest.

This can't be happening to me right now. No way. This is not my journey. I am going to

get pregnant, and this will all go away.

This is not real.

I was pregnant at eighteen. I can get pregnant!

The timing must be off. That has got to be it.

Maybe it is the wine.

Maybe God hates me.

Instead of feeling excited about this next step, I was worried. I felt like I was in the reject

pile, but I was still willing to try.

I wasn't sure if my husband should be there for the first infertility treatment, us holding hands and gazing into each other's eyes. I remember vividly tucking the semen tube into my hot-pink sports bra to keep the little guys alive with the heat of my body as I sped to the hospital. I even imagined being pulled over by the cops for rolling through a stop sign, showing him my semen tube, and yelling at him, "DO YOU SEE WHAT THIS IS? I'VE GOT SEMEN IN MY BRA,

AND I'M ON MY WAY TO THE HOSPITAL TO GET AN IUI! I HAVE GOT TO GO NOW, NOW, NOW!"

While sitting in rows of navy blue waiting chairs, with paintings of wildflower landscapes on the walls, I stared at all the pregnant women glowing with excitement to see their miracle baby on the ultrasound and hear the little heartbeat. Some had two or three toddlers running wild in the waiting room, pulling all of the toys out of the kid basket, waving at me, and occasionally saying hello as children do to strangers. It was something I longed for and could envision being a part of. Did any of the pregnant ones have trouble like me? I so wanted to be in their shoes.

Was I the only infertile woman sitting in this room? I watched non-pregnant women as they came and went. Was there some sort of way I could recognize whether or not they were one with me, full of bad eggs, or none at all? I guess all I was looking for was worry in the eyes, but then again, what woman enjoys going for a yearly check-up anyway? Unfortunately for me, infertility treatments happened in the same office as my regular OB-GYN office, so ordinary fertile people surrounded me.

That first infertility treatment was an intrauterine insemination (IUI), which is a procedure timed with ovulation where the semen is placed directly inside your uterus to help healthy sperm get closer to the egg. As I waited for my name to be called, I could feel the Void swirling around. The worry was keeping the Void close to me.

Remember the movie *Ghost*? Every time a bad character died, this black cloud would rise up from the ground with evil music and take the bad guy down into hell. This is what I sensed following me. The Void is a black, suffocating blob that wants nothing but the worst for you. It is made of negative energy and feeds on pain. The pain can be overwhelming and physical to the chest, bending and pulling in your heart center—tightness in the being that begets panic inside the mind.

I learned a great deal about this later. However, on this day, I still had hope, but I was aware of the Void lurking. I was not letting it in.

I didn't get pulled over, and my husband wasn't with me for the grand moment.

After waiting for what seemed like an hour, my name was finally called. As I laid my head back on the paper-lined exam table with my feet up in the stirrups, I waited patiently as the nurse practitioner pulled back and filled the syringe with the semen. I was nervous and excited at the possibility of conception happening at that very moment. Then, just like that, the nurse inserted the syringe, and the deposit was made in a matter of moments. I lay on the table for twenty minutes or so, and that was that.

Fourteen days later, I was pregnant. I was filming a Toyota commercial in San Francisco. I was a production manager in the film industry, back when we used film. I was in charge of managing the crew, housing and transportation, renting film equipment, making sure we stayed on budget, and serving as liaison of all communications for the crew and vendors. I was the first on set and the last to leave.

I wasn't sure what I was feeling, but I was peeing a lot more, my boobs hurt, and I was spotting. I refused to take a test until I got home. I was so nervous about miscarrying that I didn't want to know whether I was pregnant or not. I worried hard about the spotting and spent my time reading on the internet about the possibility of not miscarrying with spotting. In my hotel room, I took a long bath, and as I floated in the water, I held my hands over my belly and whispered encouragement to my unborn child.

It is safe, little one; we can do this.

I knew I was pregnant.

When I returned home, I finally took the test, and there were the two lines I had longed for. I sat down on the white tiled floor and cried happy tears of joy. I was spotting off and on, so failure was still there, but I could at least revel in the present moment that I was pregnant. I was so excited that my heart felt like it might beat out of my chest. What a wonderful feeling compared to the sorrow this same bathroom had brought so many months before. I took a picture of the stick and sent it to my husband.

He called immediately. "Is that for real?"

"Yes, can you believe it? This is actually going to work out." I was beside myself with joy, walking around in circles holding the stick, and smiling.

"I love you," I told him.

"I knew it would all be okay. Love you too, be home soon." I could tell from his gentle voice that he was relieved just as much.

I am truly a woman now. I can bring forth creation in line with my birthright and out of the dark shadows of the Void. I sat in the morning sun that day on the steps of my patio leading down to the yard. My eyes were closed and I basked in the sunlight when I heard these words in my head: *I am free. I am free. I am free.* At this moment, I felt peace. In between these words, my mind rested, silent as the rays of light filled my soul. I can still feel this moment in my heart.

Later that day, the spotting turned into bleeding, and a week later, the miscarriage was done. I was eight weeks pregnant. As quickly as the light came in, it left, leaving room for the darkness of the Void to take its place. *I am not free.*

I walked barefoot around my house in a daze, not knowing how to feel, not knowing what to do until I found myself standing in the guest room that I planned to turn into the nursery. Then, the tears came falling down as I turned and slammed the door. All I could do was aimlessly walk from room to room. My emotions went from over-the-moon elation to utter disappointment in one day. There was nothing anyone could say to make it all go away.

I could not stop crying. I sat on the wood floor of my kitchen, leaning against the cabinets, arms crossed to hold myself, as I cried to my husband over the phone. He was away visiting friends in Seattle at the time.

We sat on the phone without words, mostly until I could muster something to say.

"I just can't do this. It's so hard," I blubbered.

"I know, babe. I know. Do you want me to come home?"

"No." And then he sat with me on the phone as I quietly sobbed in between my tiny, short breaths.

One of the life lessons my grandfather taught me was to never depend on a man for anything. While I took that idea literally, what he really meant was never to let a man define who you are, and that I was strong enough to take care of myself emotionally and financially. There was no reason for John to come back to town to watch me cry in the corner. There was nothing he could do or say to help me in that moment. I needed to be alone.

For some odd reason, I took a picture of my sad face. I often look back at that photo and can feel the sadness of how I felt through the look in my sullen eyes. It was a complete reflection of the Void taking over. The Void was now inside my body, looking out at me through my own eyes. I had allowed the blob to enter and suffocate my heart. I will never forget this moment. I was devastated because I believed that I had won the struggle with this pregnancy, that I was free and no longer had to be in a state of worry, panic, and failure, only to find myself engulfed in all of it. This is the Void. Peace cannot live in the same space.

I wanted to be part of the universal truth of living, procreation, and birthing new life because that's what we are supposed to do. That is what we are here to do. We are taught this through social conditioning. The program of my unconscious mind.

How can I be a woman if I can't have a baby?

How will I fit in with the rest of society?
What will I talk about at barbecues?

The ache in my heart was signaling to me that a large and looming life lesson was at my doorstep. Life was coming for me, but I was not ready to listen.

Since I could conceive, the doctors wanted me to try again with IUI. IUI number two was not successful. For the third round, we tried a low-stimulation drug, also known as Gonadotropin, that is used to help the ovaries stimulate more than one follicle, therefore increasing the chances for conception.

Just reading that word was intimidating; gonad what? Not to mention the "how to give yourself a shot in the stomach" speech I got in the doctor's office. In the exam room, the doctor pulled out a bag of needles and showed me how to fill up the syringe with the meds.

Then she said, "Just count to three, and on three, stab away."

My eyes were as big as saucers. I had never given myself a shot. But I guess a shot in the belly, the fattest part of the body, was the best location. When it came time for me to do it, I sat at the breakfast nook in my kitchen, loaded the syringe with the meds, squeezed my belly fat between my thumb and first finger, and then froze. The needle was about an inch long but not very thick.

I am supposed to stab myself in the belly with this?

I counted, one, two, nope. I did it again, one, two, hell nope. Then finally, on the third try, I squinted my eyes almost closed and jabbed the needle through my skin. To my surprise, it really didn't hurt.

Using this new drug gave me hope. It seemed I could beat the odds by producing more than one egg each month.

This is going to work. I can feel it.

The hope was alive for this new protocol. After all, I was willingly stabbing myself in the gut each cycle. It has to work this time.

"Believe it, and it will be," Hope whispered.

Two more IUIs later, it was clear that this part of the protocol was a bust for my body. Every month for six months, I would lay on the table with my feet up in the stirrups and stare at the monitor as we looked for my eggs on day eleven or twelve. Like clockwork, there he or she would be, floating on the screen, waiting for the tadpoles. I could still ovulate eggs each month, and with John's superior sperm (all his tests showed no issues), the connection wasn't happening. It was mind-boggling to me. There is the egg. There is the sperm swimming around close together. Why won't the sperm jump in there?

The Void was growing stronger, expanding its presence inside my body. It had a tight hold on my heart, and the pressure was inseparable from my being.

"More fear. More panic. This is what I need," said the Void.

I was feeling anxious, desperate, and fat.

Toward the end of year one of the infertility treatments and two years of trying to conceive, I had completed all the IUIs that I could handle. My husband and I met with the doctors one last time. We sat in silent failure as we waited for Dr. Pimento.

"Well, we have done all the treatments we can provide you. You can continue to do IUIs if you decide, but if conception hasn't happened by now, it won't work. We suggest trying in vitro fertilization as your next step."

I took a deep breath of defeat as my shoulders collapsed. She handed us a bunch of papers, and we left. Neither of us had much to say on the car ride home. I gazed out the window, unsure if I had enough energy to blink as I processed what we had to do next.

John grabbed my hand, "You okay?" I loved his smooth hands. His touch was gentle and caring.

I squeezed back. "I'm just sad and wish we didn't have to do all of this."

"But we do have to do this. So let's go do it," he said matter-of-factly but with kindness in his voice and care in his hazel eyes.

As I stared out the window, I remembered his mother's story when I told his parents we were having issues. I knew they were wondering why I wasn't pregnant yet. I didn't talk much with his family about what we were going through. I felt awkward about sharing what seemed like our sex life with them.

We sat on the wooden benches around our kitchen table, drinking our morning coffee together.

"I am sure you are wondering when we plan to start a family," I offered.

"Why yes, we have been curious," she said respectfully.

"Well, we are having a problem, and it doesn't look like we can conceive naturally, so we are in treatment."

There was silence in between thoughts.

"You know, I was told that I could never have children because of my severe scoliosis." We both smiled because she had given birth to three ten-pound boys. My mother-in-law was about five foot three, although she would tell you she would be much taller without her back scrunch. So, to produce three huge babies in her condition was a miracle.

Then she said, "I always dreamed of riding to the hospital on my way to give birth, and then one day with your John, it happened, and it will happen for you."

This brought tears but more for the hope of the dream. Ever since this share, while riding in cars to treatments, I often found myself drawing on this story and imagining I was going to the hospital to have my baby. I tried to imagine what the feeling of the moment would be— the excitement, the worry, and the joy of having a baby. This helped get me through the pain.

What was happening to me with each treatment failure was that my belief system was being compromised and challenged, but I was unaware this was unfolding for me. I could not see it. I was raised with the idea that I can do anything. Dream it, wish for it, manifest it, and I can create the life I want. Throughout my childhood, this was repeated to me by my Grandaddy. We would spend hours together at the golf course, me driving the cart, barely able to reach the pedal. It was here that he taught me the secrets of the world. But when I could not get pregnant, my world came crashing down.

You can do anything—except have a baby.

Chapter 2

The Big Leagues

"A bend in the road is not the end of the road...
unless you fail to make the turn."

HELEN KELLER

I was feeling sad and dejected from all of the failed IUIs. I had so much hope that we would succeed through at least one of them! From all the work we had put into the procedures and tests and tests and more tests, the letdown to walk away from those tries empty-handed was devastating. But there were other options, and I was grateful that we even had another option. After all, there was still hope for us, plus I had spent time reading about the countless success stories online. Why couldn't I be one of those success stories?

Deep in the throws of treatment, it was a no-brainer to make the decision to advance to the big leagues and try in vitro fertilization (IVF). IVF is the joining of the sperm and the egg in a petri dish, a.k.a. fertilization outside the body. I still could not believe this was our fate. I had imagined getting pregnant as soon as we committed to starting a family. That is how it worked for all of my friends, so I thought the same thing would happen to me. And then when it didn't, I could not get past the disbelief that this was not going to happen naturally. That's the part Hope plays in all of this: that I might become one of the lucky ones and conceive out of the blue, in between treatments! This is what I secretly wished for, and I was counting on the Grandaddy lessons to work for me here.

At that point in time, IVF procedures were not offered in Montana. The closest place was Seattle, but we decided on Philadelphia since my cousin (not blood-related) had success there. They were considered "high FSH" friendly, which was my official diagnosis. "High follicle-stimulating hormone" is indicative of perimenopause. This meant I was running out of eggs and not the ideal IVF clinic candidate. As it turns out, creating humans is a money maker, and success rates are the main focus.

I was not afraid of "going under" for egg retrieval. I looked forward to this part of the experience, which was necessary for the egg retrieval. As my eyes became heavy, my body relaxed and let go of the stress it had been carrying. It was the only amount of peace I had experienced in over ten months. Apparently, when I first came to and they wheeled me back to my room through the maze of hallways, I looked at the nurses as I drew my words out long, "Hey, hey…what I neeeeeeeeeeed are enchilaaaaaaadas and margaritaaaaaaas. Who's with me?" This made them giggle. But I wasn't done. "And you know what? I am taking all of you with me for my interview on Oprah after the success of my one egg transfer."

Yes, that's right, I had one egg, compared to the norm of ten to fifteen. The struggle is real, like real, real.

The prep work in the month before the IVF procedure was extremely intense, filled with blood draws every other day at the hospital, plus ultrasounds to monitor egg production and growth so the doctors could best measure how many cubic centimeters (cc's) of hormones to inject in my belly. The timing of it all was crucial to success. Every second of this process was overwhelming and led by fear of failure from missing the tiniest window of time in the moment of ovulation. This fear was all-encompassing in my soul because this procedure was the last straw for me. If this didn't work, I was out. I would not be doing any more treatments.

Unknowingly at the time, I put a huge amount of pressure on myself to succeed. But this is my very nature: to win at all costs. When I was a little girl, my Grandaddy taught me this concept.

"You got to remember to keep your eye on the prize," he said to me while driving me home from Houston where he lived to my hometown in Dallas. I spent my summers with my grandparents, and he drove the five hours to pick me up and take me back home. I was riding in the back seat on the couch in the light tan Dodge van, with my feet on the windows, chewing bubble gum.

Keep your eye on the prize, I repeated to myself. I did not know exactly what this meant.

"Grandaddy, what do you mean? What prize?" I asked him.

"Well, it is when you want something really bad, but you have to work hard for it to get it. Like learning how to ride a bike. You wanted to learn how to ride that bike and tried for an entire day and didn't quit till you got it. That's what it means to keep your eye on the prize." He said.

The will to succeed was planted that day from my Grandaddy. The pressure I put on myself through negative self-talk—*You are a failure if you can't get pregnant. What will you do with your life without children? You will have nothing if this doesn't happen*—created stress that my mind simply could not handle. The only coping skill I knew was to block out all the thoughts to stop any emotion so I could get through the day. But the pressure proved too great, and it was hard to hold the emotion down. This only fueled my emotional outbursts to come, as the stress was significant and overwhelming.

I honestly don't know how my husband handled my mood swings during this time. I was wild-eyed on crazy hormones, and any little thing was rocking me from what little center I had left, sending me from a quiet whisper to yelling at the top of my lungs about something stupid like folding the towels wrong. I was not myself, and he just hung tight as much as possible, saying little during these outbursts for fear of what explosion of emotions would come out of me.

But he still was my greatest supporter, even through the tantrums. He was kind and would sit with me when I cried. He would put his arms around me and tell me, "It is all going to work out. Just give it time." He was there for any appointment when I needed him to be and gave me the space to sit in my emotions. He was always there on the sidelines, there to hold my hand when I needed it most, doing his best to bring me comfort.

I will never forget walking through the hallways of the Philadelphia clinic during our visit the day before the retrieval, past the IVF "man room" where he would have to produce on demand. I saw the ordinary vanilla room, furnished with a plaid seventies orange and green fabric-covered armchair, television, and porno videos resting on a side table with a box of tissues. The vibe was creepy just knowing all the husbands that had come before.

And there's the jack-off room.

I could only imagine the look on his face when the IVF staff guided him to that room and left him there.

The night before the retrieval was the most intense. We were "told" to have sex before we went to sleep, and then at two o'clock in the morning, my husband had to inject the human chorionic gonadotropin (hCG) shot into my ass. The hCG hormone is what tells the body to ovulate. Once given, then the retrieval of the egg can happen. Even though I had been injecting myself in the belly for over the past few months, for some reason, the idea of bending over and letting my husband stab me with a gigantic three-inch needle freaked me out.

After we left the clinic, we went out for dinner. Tomorrow was the big day, and my anxiety seemed lighter, knowing that we were almost there. The anticipation had been building for weeks, but with the moment so close, I felt strangely calm.

"You good with the shot part?" I asked. I was worried that he would hit my hip bone, lose our only hCG, and ruin the whole cycle. We had too much on the line—the procedure, airline tickets, hotels, hospital visits, thousands of dollars on hormones and procedures, not to mention the time and stress of getting this far—all to get our baby in our arms.

I could tell he wasn't sure how to answer as he mulled over how to respond. "I'm not too excited about it, but I know I can do it if that's what we must do."

Gulp.

"Well, did you ever have to give shots to cattle on the feedlot in Nebraska?" Surely he had, and we could use this as encouragement.

"Yes. And those were huge needles."

"Okay then, imagine my ass is a heifer, and stab it," we laughed in disbelief that this is what our baby-making experience had come to.

We continued to discuss the event's timing, much like a review of a business itinerary. I told him, "Let's go to bed early; I'll set the alarm for one forty-five o'clock in the morning, sex at two o'clock in the morning, and then the shot." We both sat in the restaurant with half smiles, looking at each other in silent hope. There it finally was again.

Before we knew it, two o'clock in the morning was here. We had our non-romantic planned sex, and then we got ready for the shot. We marked the spot on my butt with a marker. Both of us had our eyes wide open and we looked so unsure. I grabbed hold of the bathroom counter, bent over, and waited.

"What's going on back there?" I asked.

"Well, I'm nervous. Just give me a second," he said.

Crap.

I waited for five minutes. We were missing the window.

"You just gotta do it. Don't think," I instructed.

"Okay, okay, I know, I know," he said more to himself than to me. "Let's count it off then."

So we counted together: "One, two…." Before we got to "three," he jabbed the needle into my butt and injected the hCG perfectly.

I turned and looked at him, "I thought we said three?"

"I never do it on three. Look, it's done, right?" he hugged me, "Let's go back to bed."

Then we cuddled. As we drifted off to sleep, I felt peaceful for the first time in a long time.

All went as perfectly planned as possible. The egg fertilized beautifully, and the cells were dividing as expected, with only a tiny spot of fragmentation, so not one hundred percent perfect, but good enough to get 2AA as the grade, one being the best. My parents drove their motorhome up to visit, so we hung out in the motorhome and watched *Wyatt Earp*, which was playing as a marathon stretch on CMT the whole week we were in Philly. We named our one baby egg Wyatt. Seemed fitting. The clinic gave us a photo of Wyatt, eight cells old, that I still keep in my underwear drawer.

During this entire process, I was not relaxed. My energy was frantic, like I had not been able to sleep for days and was trying to function with zero sleep. I constantly checked my temperature, and my email for updates from the clinic. I was fidgety and locked in worry, like a strung-out drug addict on the streets. I would have emotional outbursts over what to eat for dinner. I did not stop once to try and connect with the joy in the process. It never even crossed my mind.

The positive is that we had a chance that these treatments might work. But I overlooked that part, thanks to the Void blocking me from my power. My power to connect with my courage and strength. Instead, I was entirely focused on not losing my shit. To me, this was it. I only had enough in me to do this procedure once. Even though I read stories from countless women who had done it three, five, or even ten times before they were successful, I could not bring myself to go through it again. I was not happy with the woman I was through treatment. I did not like her. She was erratic in her behavior and freaking out over everything. I did not like the way this experience made me feel, and I was exhausted emotionally. That, and the running out of eggs part. The reason why I wanted to do IVF was so that I could prove to myself that I tried everything to get pregnant. I held my breath for two weeks.

There was a lot of hope in those two weeks because I had the picture. I had proof that the connection was made, and baby Wyatt was in my womb, floating around. As we approached day fourteen, I felt energy moving around in my uterus. Was this implantation cramps or my period getting ready to come on? I went to the bathroom and saw a light spot.

Crap.

The next day, my period came on full when I woke up in the morning.

There I was again, in my bathroom. I was more than deflated. I stared at myself in the mirror for a long time. No thoughts now, only defeat. My green eyes were tired. My brown hair was messy, and I was borderline rocking the homeless vibe.

This is over. You did your best, and the dream is dead.

I went for a hike with my dogs and held on to nothing.

Needless to say, I thought that I was at the bottom of the ocean before IVF, but now I was buried in it. My heart was cold and forgotten.

The pain in my chest was expanding and hard. I couldn't breathe from the pressure of it all.

The Void had won. It had completely taken over every cell in my body. Later that night, I opened a bottle of wine, lay on my basement floor, listened to the song "Don't Panic" (a song by Coldplay), and tried to think through the pain again.

Well, fuck this. I was never meant to have kids. Why did I try anyway? I am done with this.

Gone was the happy girl I used to be, full of life and inspiration, forever marked, forever changed. Where was she? How could I get her back? I couldn't even conjure up a smile.

There I would sit at dinner parties with nothing to contribute to the conversation. I was nowhere to be found. What was there to smile about? I was an outsider everywhere. No one in my circle was experiencing this. This was a new kind of loneliness, and that's what kills you—the lack of connection with anyone. And the isolation was unbearable.

How do I get out of this? What is the answer?

I had no answers. I was no longer in control of my emotions. They were in control of me, with panic being the loudest. The sensation of fear this presented in me only provided overwhelming feelings of anxiety. My heart carried the weight of mud, and my mind was lost in pain.

I cannot have children.

The dream is over.

My life is nothing.

Chapter 3

Healed but Still Broken

**"You are headed for a breakdown.
Why don't you pull yourself to pieces."**

GROUCHO MARX

The healer came into my life through my aunt and uncle. The healer was Carl, an old family friend of theirs who was intuitive, both medically and spiritually. Some might say psychic, but to me, he was a healer. He traveled across the country, treating horses and people along the way with delicate chiropractic touches, using his energy and vision to tune into the pain of both the animals and the humans. He had a great ability to see into the emotions and help release any blockages in the body, to move stuck energy to bring healing. It was just something he innately knew.

A week after the failed IVF, my aunt called from Texas.

"It didn't work," I cried to my aunt over the phone. As fate would have it, the healer was visiting. They had come in for lunch after treating the horses, and Carl was listening at the kitchen table as my aunt talked with me.

When she hung up the phone, he asked her, "What happened to the left side of her body?"

Surprised that he could know this, my aunt said, "Well, she hit a tree with that side while snowboarding."

"Well, her uterus is tilted and off-center. Her ribs are compacted there, and her body cannot conceive."

She called me back immediately. "Get down here now. Carl says it was the accident, and the damage to your body is the problem. He is here and can help you."

Until now, I hadn't even considered this might be part of the equation. It was something so obvious, and I had questioned it in the hospital, but since I was ovulating every month like clockwork, I kept thinking that everything was working correctly. Suddenly, it was clear to me. This seemed to be the most logical explanation for my misfortune. It wasn't God damning me from the rest of the world because of some wrongdoing I did in a past life. I had hit a tree, and my body was injured.

I caught a flight out the next morning to Texas. I was open to anything and finally relieved to have something tangible that made sense to me. I could not bring myself to believe the doctors when they told me I was perimenopausal at the age of thirty-four. There is no history of this in my family, for crying out loud.

At this point, I had no expectations of how the healing would unfold, other than being open to the experience. I have seen various healers in my life. These experiences have taught me to be open to healers and their unique ways of performing their healing. Carl was a wide-chested cowboy from South Dakota. Not at all what you would imagine when you think of a healer. The first thing he had me do was walk back and forth across the living room terra-cotta tiles. With my aunt and uncle watching, he observed me intently as I walked back and forth. I wasn't sure what he was looking for, so I kept on going until he spoke.

"You see that right there?" I stood tall in front of the group, and he pointed to my knees. "The left one is higher than the right, and her left shoulder is higher than her right."

What was he talking about? I ran over to the mirror to look for myself, and I was as crooked as a dog's hind leg. "Wow, look at that," I said, turning from side to side to see the difference. I was in shock. I didn't feel crooked, nor like I was walking with a slight limp, and I wasn't in any pain at all, or so I thought.

Carl laughed, "You have been walking around like this for three years! Your body has adjusted, and what you feel now is normal to you." His eyes communicated his gentle ways as he spoke with thoughtful pause and clarity. "You see here," he pointed to my pelvis, "it is not in the right position."

While he was examining my body, my energy body was talking to him the same way the horses spoke to him. *Help me. Something isn't right in my heart.* He had a calming essence about him that was strong and engaging. In a time when no one could reach me, there was a rope of hope I saw in Carl as he threw it down for me to catch. I was so deep in the Void that it took everything I had to hang on.

"Do you really think this is going to help get me pregnant?"

"Yes, I do. Your body is not balanced," Carl could see.

"I still can't believe I never checked my injury with a chiropractor. How did I not think of this till now?" I asked.

"Because the doctors should have told you and didn't."

My healer was not only a chiropractor but a body and energy reader. He has the ability to tune into the body and touch the heart, gut, and mind, the three intricate designs of the soul, with his healing energy. How he does this, I have no idea.

Lying on my aunt's bed surrounded by rustic Western motifs, I took in a couple of deep breaths. I had so much pain in my chest. If I breathed deep enough, would it get out? I stared intently at Carl as he gathered himself with deep breaths of his own. *Trust him.* He rubbed his hands together, then, with his eyes closed, he ran his hands a few inches over my body from head to toe and back to the center. He focused on my uterus, around my hips, and my ribs, where the memory of the injury still lived.

Next, he pulled out his tools, a tiny hammer and a chisel. "I'm going to work on your pelvic bone here on the left side, which will help even out the length of your legs. Then, I'm going to focus on your ribs. The way both of these areas are resting is making it nearly impossible to conceive. Even if by some miracle you were to conceive and carry to twenty-five weeks, the way your ribs are stuck together, they would keep your body from expanding properly. After this adjustment, we will rest, as your body is going to be sore," he told me.

Then, much like a woodworker carving a flower, he manipulated my pelvis, pubic bones, and ribs. It was a tapping sensation. Sometimes a rapid tap, and other times one hard tap to snap the bones in place. I felt a release after each tap, much like what you feel when you crack your neck or your back when you roll your shoulders back around in a circle.

I was in awe of what he was telling me. Finally, someone offered some positive information on my infertility journey that made sense. After he hammered on my bones, he then took his big cowboy hands and massaged my organs deeply, specifically my spleen, small intestine, and uterus. It felt like his hands were inside my body, rearranging these organs back to the proper location.

Then we were done. There was no magic spell Carl cast over my body and no prayer to the healing gods above; we were simply done. "We will rest for now, and I will do this same procedure tomorrow. Let's let the body do the rest."

The next day, I could barely get out of bed. My body felt like I had hit the tree all over again. Carl repeated the same technique as before, and with each tap, I could feel the Void grow more agitated—it would squeeze my lungs in response to the adjustments, digging down into my heart to maintain control there. The energy of the healing was coming for it, and it knew it. Because the healing energy was positive and of hope, the Void cannot live in this energy. After Carl finished, this time, we were not done. There was more.

He took a deep breath and said, "I'm going to do something with your body, and I may have to run out of the room and get sick. I don't want you to be alarmed."

I guess this mystical moment was what I had been waiting for in the healing. He closed his eyes and ran them all over the top of my body, much like how we started the healing the day before, and then he brought them back to my heart. He concentrated on this area, and I knew exactly what he was doing. I could feel his energy transfer to mine as it swirled around the part that needed to be removed. I breathed in and out deeply as I released the Void onto him. From the core of my being, I pushed it all out as hard as I could. I wanted to be free of this feeling of suffocation that I had been carrying for so long. All of a sudden, Carl ran out of the room, and I could hear him vomiting in the bathroom.

I lay there for a good twenty minutes, lighter in my chest, completely mesmerized by what I had experienced, yet surprised that I felt calm inside. The frantic energy of panic had subsided. I did not feel healed from the pain I had been carrying—there were still scars there to heal—but I did feel better. I no longer felt suffocation. It had left my body and was replaced with the light energy of hope. Carl came back into the room to check on me, "How do you feel?"

"What was that? Are you okay?" I wanted to make sure the Void didn't jump on him. I think he was amused that I was concerned for him, the healer.

"I'm fine. That was why I got sick right after. I had to get that out of you and make sure it did not stay with me. Sometimes that happens," he said with a wide smile.

Even though I knew what "it" was, I wanted to know how he saw it, "What was 'it' like?" I asked.

"I felt it there yesterday. It was very strong and extremely negative. It had a hold of you. It felt like black goo. It was so strong, I wasn't sure if I would be able to get it, but today it jumped right out onto me."

I smiled and laid my head back on the pillow as this feedback validated my feelings about the Void. On some level, something needed to shift in me to get rid of it. You know, when we are depressed about something and it takes over our life, this allows the negative. The Void wins and cuts off the joy in our life. It thrives on cutting us off from the good parts of life, happiness, and the beauty of all that is. As it takes over, and we slide deeper and deeper into the hole, we feel as if no one else can understand, probably because we can't even understand ourselves. Who wants to sit around having cocktails after work while listening to me talk about my emotional problems? But when we are in the thick of life's greatest lessons, the hardship is all-encompassing. When it takes over, we disconnect from others, a huge victory for the Void.

Carl and I spent the rest of that day talking, heart to heart. It was a necessary part of the healing because my heart had been shut down, and he was opening it back up, petal by petal. "You will be a mother, Shannon. I can see it. You have to believe in it."

He paused before opening his heart fully to me, " I have had pain too." As we stood outside in the late afternoon, he looked deeply into my eyes as I hung onto every word, "My daughter was killed in a car wreck at eighteen, and I knew it when she left the house. I looked at her, and all I could see was red. It was the most difficult experience of my lifetime. After living through the grief, I realized that I had a choice either to let this tragedy have my life or to continue to live through it and find peace. Even though my heart was broken and there will always be a piece of me forever changed by this, I still had to make this choice. We all do at one time or another, and this is the choice you have to make in your own heart now. You are not what your mind is telling you. You don't have to listen to it."

He asked me what I saw on the horizon. "Look out there and tell me what you see."

I looked across my aunt and uncle's thirty acres. "I see green pastures lined with mesquite trees against the Texas blue sky." But I kept searching past that. "I see a haze above the tree line, like a desert mirage of orange light." *Do I now have special powers and am seeing a vision from beyond?* It was as if the healing had given me some sort of special sight.

But the reality was much different. "Really? That's what you see?" I looked at him while questioning myself, "Yes, that's what I see." But I was unsure. "I think."

"You think," he said to me and then stared right through me.

I darted my eyes around, not sure where this was headed. *That's what I thought I saw.* There was silence, then more silence. I smiled. This was uncomfortable.

He softened, "What is on the horizon are trees and blue sky. That's it, nothing more or less. You have been going from here (he put his hand on my head) to here (put his hand on my heart), when you need to be going from gut to heart to head. Hear from the belly first."

What, my head had been running the show this whole time?

The fear was coming from my mind. The hard part about infertility is that with each cycle of the moon, each spot of blood, the dream ends only to begin again. With each passing cycle, the mind begins to catch on and feed the Void. *Nope. Not this month. Strike forty-two.* Sometimes, I could get through a month without the diatribe of the mind. But more than likely, it goes something like this: *You see. You are not going to be a mother. You are not good enough. You can't do it. Your body is broken.*

You are broken. Give up. It's never going to happen for you. How long are we going to keep doing this? This is what it felt like each month as I stared in the mirror and cried my eyes out in my sacred bathroom, which wasn't much of a bathroom. It was a basement bathroom, simple and white, with red towels. There were no windows, and the floor was cold, lined with white tiles. No one could hear me down there.

The Native Americans of the plains of South Dakota referred to Carl as the White Horse. They accepted him as a true medicine man, even as a white man. I learned so much from this healing. He taught me to tap into the wisdom from within. To hear the messages from my gut first.

The next month, I got pregnant. It just happened. No more shots, no bloodwork, no infertility treatments, no pills, no acupuncture, no temperature monitors, no organic everything food; hell, I didn't even know what day of the month I was having sex on. As much as I hate to say it, the one time I truly let go and thought about nothing, I conceived. The idea of "just let it go, and it will happen" still pisses me off. How can I let go when I have to schedule doctor appointments, get blood draws, take my temperature every day, chart my ovulation, and time sex? I have to plan and think to schedule all of this. It is very hard to "let go" and sit back and relax. To me, "let go" means be carefree, don't worry about it, and it will happen when it happens. Let go of the panic. Let go of the outcome. Let go of the control. What can I not control here? I can't control when another life comes in. It is not our choice; it is the baby's choice. We are merely the portal through which they come through.

My hormone numbers were doubling every day, and the first ultrasound was good. I truly felt blessed. This conception was a gift and showed me that the healer was real. As I walked from the parking garage down Main Street to my office one day, I found myself in a new inner calmness while waiting on the corner to cross the street. This was the first pregnancy I felt this. My mind was quiet and free of worry. I got this one this time. This one is here to stay. I laid my hand over the jellybean in my belly. *Keep your heart open.*

My mother and I are very close, almost like sisters, and we talk daily. She was and has always been my rock, knowing me like no other human. Naturally, I leaned on her the most as I processed.

"Mom, it all looks good. The hormones show progression. I feel pregnant, my boobs hurt, and my womb feels a little achy."

"Good. This is all that it should be. When's the ultrasound?" she asked.

"Next week. We will get to hear the heartbeat next!" All the boxes were getting checked off the list per each doctor visit. Getting the heartbeat was the next big confirmation for us.

Since I was considered high-risk, the doctors monitored me every week. During the ultrasound of week seven, we watched the monitor intently while the doctor searched for the embryo. It was there, but the sac was measuring a little small, and there was no heartbeat. But there was still time for the heartbeat. As I lay on the examination table, I observed the doctors like a hawk to try and read their emotions, if any. Because of my history, I didn't think they believed that I could carry to term and had already written me off as the poor reject trying to make it back into the norm pile. But I refused to listen to that. I was pregnant with a miracle baby, and this was going to happen!

I'll admit, the no heartbeat part caused me to hold my breath for an entire week. But by the following week, there it was, a tiny blip of light on the screen. I smiled as I watched the rhythm, holding John's hand. *This dream was finally coming true. I will be a Mommy. We will be Mom and Dad.*

I called my Mom on the way home. "It's there. The heartbeat is there." I could not stop smiling. This was the happiest day of my life.

"I just knew it would happen for you," she replied, and I could hear her happiness too. Happy for a grandchild, but happier that I was at peace.

John had a meeting and could not be there for the next week's appointment. This was routine, and I expected nothing more than positive news. I put on the hospital gown and positioned myself on the examination table, lined with paper that reminded me of butcher paper. The doctor rubbed warm gel on my belly and applied the ultrasound probe to my womb. A stillness filled the room. I was holding my breath. The jellybean was still there. But there was a shift in the doctor's demeanor as her eyes looked down, and there was no smile. I looked back and forth between her and the monitor, anticipating her response. "There's the sac," she said. "But nothing has changed in the last week. I'm sorry." Everything came crashing down.

The heartbeat was gone. There was no growth. It was done. I stared blankly at the monitor as the tears swelled in my eyes and my heart slowly crumbled. Over the course of a week, I went in for two more ultrasounds because I was in denial that it was actually over. Surely, they were missing the heartbeat during the scan. If we kept searching, I just knew we would find it. The nurses were annoyed at this waste of time for them. They knew the pregnancy was done, and they were merely going through the motions as long as I was willing to pay for the visits. Finally, I surrendered to the inevitable. I scheduled the DNC procedure within the next week, and the jellybean remains were sucked away from my womb.

I called Carl to let him know the pregnancy had failed. I could hear his disappointment and disbelief in his response of silence to my news. *Great, now my healer doesn't even know what to think about my uterus. I'm fucked.*

Oddly, I was not as disheartened as I was from the failed in vitro fertilization procedure. I was something different, comfortably numb.

The only thing I knew to do at this moment was shut down all of my emotions, like drawing a black curtain closed over my hardened heart as I vanished into it. There would be no more crying. There would be no more wanting. There would be no children.

The black blob of the Void had returned to my body, taking its place in my heart, smothering every part of me, just as it had before the healing. I didn't even have the strength to keep it out. There is nothing harder than the emotion of loss. The reality is that I had no choice but to face everyday glimpses of motherhood as a witness to a mother holding her child's hand, wiping snot from his nose, and hearing them call her Mommy. Knowing the closest I would ever come to this was only in a heartbeat. This brought complete devastation to my life. I had no place in society. My dream of family was shattered. Why did my baby choose to stay in Heaven? How will I ever find my way back to the peace I found on the mountain that day?

Chapter 4

In Sickness and in Health

"A perfect marriage is just two imperfect
people who refuse to give up on each other."

KATE STEWART

The likelihood of having a baby with my husband was starting to look grim. It just might be that this lifetime was meant to be about the two of us. All of our focus was on accomplishing the goal of pregnancy, but as the goal was denied over and over again, all of a sudden, it happened: we found ourselves in a marriage just coasting—not fighting, not ignoring, but existing, cohabitating.

Damn it.

Underneath it all, I harbored resentment toward him as I felt like he never dealt with the pain and simply ignored it all. I know what I did not want: a divorce to ruin my entire life because we couldn't have a baby.

I was planning on leaving out this section entirely from the book. Why are you leaving out the most important piece of the lesson? *Because I don't want to deal with it.* Ironic when my silent resentment toward him was because I felt like he wasn't dealing with it.

In the beginning of us, we used to spend our evenings driving country back roads at sunset with the windows rolled down, the wind blowing my hair in my face, a six-pack of beer, and listening to our favorite music. We weren't even engaged yet; life was carefree. I can still see us smiling, my hand dolphin-diving outside the window, singing our favorite country song by Don Williams, "I Believe in You." When I heard his words, *I believe in love, I believe in babies, I believe in Mom and Dad, and I believe in you,* I knew right then and there that this was our song, and John believed it too. We danced to this song on our wedding night in that old barn lit with tiny white lights. We smiled and looked into each other's eyes, knowing that the dream we sang on those country sunset drives was now real. Through ceremony, we were committed to our connection of us, no matter what.

That's why it was so hard and shocking to go from that dream to believe in our reality of infertility. That one day, we would end up being a statistic from a long list of inadequacies:

- **1 in 8** couples are struggling with infertility issues. (Yup, we were in this group.)
- **7.4 million** is the number of women between ages 15-44 in the U.S. who have difficulty getting and staying pregnant. That's 12% of all women. (#mytribe, whether I like it or not.)
- **7.5 percent** of men have reported seeing a fertility doctor at least once. (John's team.)
- **40 percent** of struggling couples are in the situation where the male partner contributes or is the cause of infertility. (#notmyguy, he has Olympic swimmers!)
- **13 percent** of female infertility is caused by tobacco and cigarette smoking. (Did smoking a pack a day in college cause this for me?)
- **6.1 million** is the number of women who suffer from polycystic ovarian syndrome. Affecting **10 percent** of women, PCOS is

the most common cause of female infertility. (I was surprised at this number, but this was not my problem.)

- **38 percent** of male infertility cases are tied to the most correctable cause, varicoceles (abnormal veins surrounding the testicles). (If only this stat was ours.)
- **85-90 percent** of infertility cases can be treated by conventional therapies like surgery or medication. (I prayed luck would put us here.)
- **3 percent** include infertility treatments like in vitro fertilization. (It was hard for me to fathom being in such a tiny percentile, when it felt so big.)
- **30 percent** is the estimated percentage of an IVF cycle producing a live birth. (#nope)
- **25 percent** of couples have more than one factor, contributing to their infertility as a pair. (Good Lord, I am glad my aging womb was the only factor—that's hard enough.)
- **20 percent** of infertility cases have no known cause. (I can't imagine a more frustrating diagnosis. If there is no reason, then why can't it just happen?)[1]

In our case, it was my body that had the issue. This means I will be the person who will cope with the failure the most, if not all. When it is your body enduring the testing, the prodding, and the poking, it's hard not to be reminded daily of the mounting pressure.

Ten years after our carefree newlywed days, I sat with John and read him an early draft of this chapter at our kitchen table. I was curious how he would perceive the words, to hear the pain again. Still today, he sat uncomfortable in his plaid shirt, unsure what this reading might lead to next. Was it out of fear of that insane person showing up? I watched him as I read aloud. He leaned forward and looked down at the ground as he listened to my words. Did he not want to hear the story anymore, or was it the sadness from the outcome we live with today? After years of not knowing, we finally had our connection talk.

"Did you feel failure during the treatments?" I asked.

Without hesitation, he answered, "No. I did not experience failure in that sense. I never felt that way."

I tilted my head and squinted my eyes in contemplation because I couldn't understand how in the hell he did not feel failure when I was buried in it.

"I just assumed that you were feeling failure like me, and we never talked about it. I guess we have never talked about how you felt." I responded, holding the crazy person down. If I let her come out now, she would end this conversation. The fact that he didn't experience failure bothered me. I guess because I felt like a failure and assumed he felt the same. I would learn that this was my hang-up with him because it made me feel that much more alone in the pain.

Under the heavy pregnancy pressure, there was no room in my heart to see the big picture of what was going on with our marriage, in how we were or weren't showing up for one another. I was focused on surviving, moving through the checklists to succeed, and doing whatever the doctors told me to do to get pregnant. Honestly, back then, if I had asked whether or not he felt failure, would I have even been able to handle him telling me he didn't? *Probably not.* Even worse, I would have used this against him as I laid another brick on the resentment wall.

"Well, what did you feel then?" I wondered.

"I felt disappointed," he said.

Oh no, do not cry here. If he sees you cry, he will clam up and think the crazy person is coming up next. But I couldn't stop the tears that welled up in my eyes when he told me this. I knew in my heart he felt this way.

I took in a breath and fought back a tear. "You felt disappointed because you would not be a father? You won't know what being a father is like?"

He was very uncomfortable and fidgeting in his chair, eyes diverting down, clearly wanting out of this conversation. He must have been wondering if this was some sort of setup.

I reached for his hand and told him, "It's okay to speak your truth, no matter how it might make me feel, even if your truth is not some pretty package of perfect. It's okay to tell me."

He looked at me with his strong hazel eyes and said, "Yes, that is it. I felt disappointed because I will never know what it is like to have my own family."

I squeezed his hand and let a few tears fall on the table. "We would have been great parents together," I smiled at him.

"Yes, we would have been," he smiled and squeezed my hand back.

He never said this to me until I asked the question, but how could he otherwise? How could he come to me and say, "You know, I am super disappointed that your body failed and we were unable to have children together and raise a family; thanks for nothing, wife." During the tough infertility moments, there is no way he could have said this to me. My mind would have only heard this as a failure, my failure.

But did he have pressure like me? I had a flashback of when we waited together in the pale-blue sterile office for the doctor to deliver the first of many test results. This one was big because we would find out whose body was broken. *Is it me or him, or will we be in the twenty percent of the unknown cases?* My FSH came back very high at 21. His sperm were normal. I could tell from his body language that a sense of relief came over him when his shoulders relaxed, and he leaned back in his chair. I would learn later that his pressure looked much different from mine.

It took me a few days to process the results. I did not want it to be him because I felt like the pressure of failure would be too much for him to handle. I honestly would rather carry that for him, in a sense. *I can handle this pressure. I've got this for us.* And just like that, I unknowingly energetically made an agreement with myself that I would carry the pressure "so he didn't have to." I made this agreement without him and blamed him for this unspoken agreement. *Welcome to the party, resentment.*

How will we stay connected through this mess? In year one of our marriage, we found ourselves in our first major life challenge. I found we bonded on being outsiders. While all of our married friends were adjusting to being new parents, learning how to live with each other, and coping with losing their independence as parents, we observed and compared our relationships with others.

These moments would come during normal social settings, like hosting a dinner party with friends. Not soon after the treatments ended, we had friends over for dinner. I was busy setting the table with our red dinner plates, a wedding gift we still used, lined with vanilla-colored napkins, John was grilling steaks. Jerry Garcia was playing "Dear Prudence" in the background. It was a nice autumn evening. Meanwhile, our guests were trying to feed their three-year-old, who was cranky and refusing to do anything. The tension was building for them. The couple was bickering quietly with each other while they fought through whose method was best. John and I caught each other's eye as we moved around in the kitchen. In this silent connection, I know we wished we could have this kind of moment together. I could feel my heart swell a little and then tighten.

Our lives were so different from everyone else because inside, we were fighting to have a family so that we could carry on like the rest of humanity. Even as outsiders, we were still "we." We were in our own unique version of togetherness, united in our special bond wrapped up in an infertility bomb.

Sometimes this bomb would just show up on any given night. Like one night, sitting in front of the fire on the ground, wrapped in my cream rosebud throw, drinking wine, contemplating everything. The warmth of the fire was comforting, but short-lived. Often, this led to my greatest meltdowns, because really what I was doing here was looking at my pain. As I reviewed all that was not working, after more sips of wine, then the anger would show up. And I needed to talk about it and get it out. This was my process.

John was sitting on the leather couch on his phone. Dogs were sleeping next to his feet—a typical night for us.

"When will I stop crying about this?" I asked him calmly. "This pressure is so great for me."

He looked up from his phone. "I don't know, babe."

"It's just so huge. I can't grasp the magnitude of what this means. I keep trying but don't know what to do with it. Do we just wait this out?" My voice was starting to shake. My heart felt like it might explode in my chest. I took a sip of wine. I was good and drunk at this point.

John was tense and worried. He knew what was coming.

"I can't be around pregnant people. I'll never get away from that ever in my life!" I yelled at him as I burst into tears.

John stared back silently.

The more he sat silent, the louder I got, slobbering, crying while trying to catch my breath, mascara all over my face, squeezing my blanket like a baby on the floor. To him, I feared I looked like a tweaked-out meth addict acting completely insane. I imagined he must be thinking, "What the hell is this? I married this sane woman, and now she has lost her fucking mind!" That's what it felt like when he calmly sat on the couch and stared back at me in silence, scared for the monster I had become. This was what my mind had convinced me was the truth.

"I'm not doing this again," he put his foot down.

On the outside, he seemed like he didn't care because he never wanted to talk about it. This would infuriate me, and I would act out even more. I would tell myself, *why would he care? This is not his problem; his body is fine.* The resentment was building. The suffering part of me walked around with tense muscles, jaw clenched, and held my breath constantly. *Good God, did I ever even take a breath?* My husband chose not to talk about it; that was his way of coping.

"I can't even talk to you when you are like this. You need to relax," he would say to me often. He didn't know what else to do or say to me. How could he? I was out of control, and the meltdowns would not stop. This alien wife was scaring the shit out of him because she was threatening our connection. We were not on the same page, and our hearts began to disconnect. This was no way to communicate.

People cope differently and in their own time, period. One cannot control another in the timing of dealing with emotional pain. On one hand, you have me slamming doors, storming out of rooms, and rolling my eyes. I thought this was me dealing with it. On the other hand, there was John, abstaining from conflict together, saying nothing, and walking away. I chose outburst; he chose to go within.

I was always struck when I heard of divorce after the death of a child. I could never understand this because I imagined that experiencing a loss of this enormity would bring you closer than ever before. But the reality is that everyone has different ways of coping, and if not communicated clearly to one another, this can lead to misunderstandings within grief.

My anger continued to grow toward him because his life went on as usual—golf with the boys, traveling, and sports—with no care in the world. How dare he keep living his life? I, on the other hand, was living in misery. How could he even smile right now? My face was permanently pinched, my eyes in a dark scowl. I wanted my life to be normal again. I wanted us to be normal again. But the pain was in the way of living my life and sharing it with John. I was not happy and not interested in anything, and I was mad at him for feeling different than this. Naturally, I had no interest in spending quality time together or paying any attention to us.

With all that said, one day while scouring the internet for relief, I read these words. "Infertility is not forever." *Say what?* The truth is, we will not be struggling to conceive one day. Infertility does have an ending. *Well, thank God for that!* But what about the aftermath? According to the National Library of Medicine, depression peaks three years post infertility. Six years post infertility, the depression and anxiety begin to fade; you start to feel stronger again. However, the healing time for couples can take much longer.[2]

Victim number one is the sex life. Infertility kills the sex life, period. There is such a thing as sexual stress, and infertility kicks that into high gear. It is a game changer in the bedroom. While in treatment or naturally trying, sex is performed on command, timed around ovulation. The male must perform in these moments. This leads to performance anxiety in the bedroom and what the male experiences as pressure. And if your sperm provider is like mine, he did not and still doesn't like to be told what to do, like ever.

I was always excited about sex because any time we had it, it could be THE time it worked. But for John, it was a command.

"Babe, this time could be the one!" I told him as I waited for him to join me in bed one afternoon.

"Uh-huh," he said while he got undressed, still looking at his work emails since he was on his lunch break. Yes, this is what we were doing: meeting at home over lunch for a quickie. He was able to perform, and he always did when asked. But he hated it. Of course, he didn't tell me then, but he did at the kitchen table during our connection talk.

"I just didn't like that pressure, to have to do it right then." And there it was, his pressure. I had the pressure of a failed uterus. He had the pressure to perform.

"Did you have resentment toward me about it?" I asked.

"No, not for you. I just knew it was the process, and that was it," he said.

What we didn't do was pay attention to our sex life outside of the trying. The entire focus was on getting pregnant, and we only had timed sex. It was not intimate. It was mechanical. Even worse, as more time went on with zero success, sex naturally felt like a failure to me. It served as a reminder that we were broken, and it sadly led to an empty sex life.

If I could redo it, I would take the time to be intimate with him, just because. Then, we might have had a chance to dissociate our trying to conceive from having sex. We did it all wrong. We left all the baby monitor crap on the bedside table—the ovulation chart and the thermometer—and every single time during sexual intimacy, I thought this could be it. That was all that was on my mind.

After countless hours of searching the internet, I read an article on how males and females experience the stress of infertility. It has been tested and measured that women experience a greater amount of stress than men do. However, both women and men are dealing with the impact of social and sexual concerns and the need for parenthood. An Oxford Academic study of attachment theory in association with couples undergoing their first IVF treatment reports that women experience the failure of treatment as extreme deterioration of emotional well-being and sex anxiety with high levels of strain on the sexual relationship.[3]

One of our screaming fights in our old brown kitchen ended up being the game changer, the moment that he got through to me, where I could hear what he was saying. Up until this point, my anger was totally taken out on him. It was another lunchtime break at home, with me screaming at how unfair this all was, when he walked out on me, slamming the door. The flower painting on the wall rattled with the slam. I just stood there breathing quick, short breaths through my nose. Then he opened the door again. "That is it!" He pointed his finger at me. "I'm tired of you yelling at me all the time. That's all you do is yell at me, and I'm sick of it. I am not the one that is causing all of this. There is nothing we can do about this. It's happening, and that is it. I am absolutely done with you treating me like shit. I am trying to be here for you, but you are making it near impossible to support you when you act like an ass." Then he left. I slid down the wall and sat on the floor, and cried. He was right. But this didn't stop my meltdowns. There were to be many more.

When John and I are connecting, we flow; it feels easy. We hang out and do the things we enjoy, like hiking, golfing, camping, music, and with a lot of laughter. It's the fun part. When I know we are most connected is how we look each other in the eyes, even in passing through the kitchen, brushing against each other, and reaching for a coffee cup. It's the same look on our wedding day: knowing we are good. It's our unspoken reassurance and commitment to us.

When we are not connecting, there is none of that. I don't even look him in the eye. I don't want to talk. I don't want to hang out. I just want to be alone until I am ready to connect. But even deeper, if I'm holding resentment, I shut him out completely. That is my coping mechanism. This I have done for a very long time and still struggle with today. In return, John shuts down and cuts me off emotionally until I have no idea what he is thinking or feeling. Coasting.

So, what's really going on here? When I focused on my inner narrative and looked at what it was telling me, I realized I was letting my thoughts take me for a ride without questioning them. *Damn it. Now we've got marriage problems. We read about this.* Infertility couples are three times more likely to divorce. *Here we go.* And when I listened to these thoughts, I began to worry. *Shit. Now, this fucking infertility is threatening my marriage because the statistics say we should be in trouble. I am at risk of having no baby and no husband.*

After infertility, I struggled with whether or not John and I were still connected. Was this idea coming from a place of without? Without a family, without children of our own to teach, without this rite of passage to connect as parents? This connection to me is a valuable piece of the relationship in learning about one another, as well as your ideals, morals, and spirituality that you would want to instill in your offspring. The raising of a family as Mom and Dad was the ultimate way to connect. Instead, we had the experience of without and learned about connection through grief and loss.

After sitting with this concept for a while, I finally heard these words.

But you still learned a lot from each other through grief and loss, like how you handled extreme stress, trauma, and sorrow. How your ideals, morals, and spirituality influenced one another as you moved through it.

While not wrapped up in a soft and cozy owl-printed baby blanket, we were still connecting through the bad news of failed procedures, miscarriages, and a not-a-mother shaming moment from that one time I was told my opinion didn't matter about child rearing because I had none. Yes, that actually happened during a ping-pong game.

We used to kid with one another about adopting an eighteen-year-old football player so we could cheer them on through college and into the NFL. We do love football, but of course, that's not a reason to adopt someone.

Years later, I was turning out the lights to go to bed, and I caught John sniffling while watching the movie *Blind Side*.

"Wait, are you crying?" I asked as I walked past his chair.

He, embarrassed, answered, "No."

In a loving way, I said, "You are crying. I see you crying." Then I put my hand on his shoulder and said, "Are you crying because this is about adopting a football player?"

He smiled. I could see somewhere in there, he hurts too. I squeezed his shoulder and went to bed. I let him have that moment privately because he needed to, and that's okay. That was his way of coping.

John and I did not process grief the same and not at the same time. I dealt with the intense pain while I was in it. I wanted to constantly analyze and talk, ahem, I mean scream my way through it. This is what I needed to get it out. If I could regurgitate all the anger my little body stored inside it, I would be left on the floor with no more emotion, a clean slate, ground zero. Then and only then could I pick myself up, start again, and grow into something new.

All I wanted was for him to hold me every single time and let me cry on his shoulder. While there were times he did this for me, there were many times he did not and left the room angry with me, like the old brown kitchen fight. But was he dealing? I felt like he wasn't. I was trying to tell him this in my meltdowns. So it only hurt me when he would shut down and say nothing, walk out of the living room, and leave me there on the floor with my dogs licking my face to deal with myself. He was telling me by walking away that I was on my own to deal with it. I could not trust that he would be there for me, so I withdrew my emotions and shut this part of me off. This is the damage that infertility causes. His walkouts ended all conversations about infertility indefinitely.

How do we reconnect? I need to challenge what I am telling myself. Instead of analyzing my relationship, I took a look at my repetitive thoughts. *What are they saying about this?* That question alone is packed with power, your superpower of awareness. *What am I telling myself, and is it true?* I got my pen and paper and began writing these thoughts down. *And what do I want?* When I challenged my inner dialogue, I found it was all about our sex life. *Why doesn't he want me anymore? Am I not beautiful enough, sexy enough, or woman enough?* I was having extreme self-esteem issues as it relates to this because none of us want to feel unwanted. This is an incredibly lonely place when your husband shows no desire or interest in you anymore. The reality is that I blame infertility for ruining our sex life. *Is this the result of our infertility stress? This is what we get? No baby, no family, and now no sex life.*

The fact that infertility left us a big shit pile of a sex life actually pissed me off. Since having a family was not an option, I will have everything else I want. I am going to have that perfect life. Then came the conversation with an old friend that challenged my idea of perfect. She said, "Wait. What is perfect anyway? Isn't it just perfect to wake up each day, to be healthy, to be breathing?" This comment stopped me in my tracks because she was right. I was holding onto the social stigma of a "perfect marriage." Two kids, a house, a couple of dogs, an amazing sex life, and a husband who adored me no matter what. That was how I defined "perfect." I actually have all those things except the kids and the amazing sex life. So, I am close to my version of perfect. He loves and adores me, but the rest is a made-up Hollywood version in my head.

So, what is "perfect" anyway? The word generally means something is completely without flaws. That is impossible for a marriage. It also means no mistakes, which is also impossible for a marriage. It means conformity to an ideal. The only way this one is possible is if you follow the social conditioning on what a marriage should look like and then lie about it to the world because there is no way that perfect Instagram marriage is for real. It's all fake as shit. What I realized is never to use the word "perfect" when describing anything in my life. It is an unattainable goal, this idea of perfection. We don't want to strive for perfection in our marriage because it is absolutely impossible. But you can strive for connection.

A deeper connection is what I really wanted from our marriage. So why can't we have sex? I was worried. But is this "without" a reason enough to leave? As I sat with this, I realized I needed to take a step back and look at all of the other intimate connections we share in our emotional and life experiences and in spiritual ways. While the lack of sexual intimacy was staring me down, I had to look at the rest to determine whether or not a relationship could survive this or not.

"Thank you for being you," I said to him often during our courting phase. This became our foundation. This phrase alone allowed us to be vulnerable, open, and accept each other for who we truly are. Intimacy is how we connect, how we communicate ourselves to each other. This is the nourishment song that we both need. Sharing emotional intimacy means that we feel safe sharing our innermost thoughts, the good and the bad.

When I stopped being mad about what infertility did to our sexual intimacy and took a look at how we connect through all levels of intimacy, from experiential to spiritual, I realized that we do have it all, almost, and we can heal the sexual intimacy that infertility stole from us.

The death of his mother, followed soon after by his father's second marriage, was an extreme amount of emotional stress for John. This came at the tail end of infertility. I knew he was struggling, and this situation had no easy fix. We had countless conversations about the emotional impact of this life change as we worked through how to process and cope with the sadness and grieving of this part of his life. This way of communicating was much easier for us than the outbursts. We can actually connect and speak this way with each other about difficult feelings.

We were experiencing life together by sharing activities like golf, camping, traveling, hiking, or country drives. These moments create memories, and memories create experiential intimacy. We have all of this.

Spiritual intimacy usually is us enjoying something breathtaking in a moment from nature, like watching eagles soar, sunsets, and full moons.

"I'm one with eagles," John proclaimed to me one summer. "I see them everywhere. It's my spirit animal." He was serious about this.

He had been outside cleaning up the yard and came running inside. "Babe, you got to come out here and see this."

"What is it?" I asked as I followed him out to the end of the driveway.

He pointed up. "Look!"

There above our house was an eagle, soaring high. His wings stretched wide as we watched him circle our house.

"It's your spirit animal coming to check you out."

"You see, I told you. They follow me now." He smiled at me.

We never miss a full moon or sunset when they are in their glory. We don't have many windows that face west in our home, so the pink glow usually lures us out to the end of the driveway. He is always up for this and joins me without hesitation. And it is John who reminds me to run outside and see the full moon. "Babe, go outside now and look at the moon." He will call me on his way home from golf. "It's amazing—you got to go see it." I always stop what I am doing and run outside, still on the phone with him, to get a glimpse. Then we stay connected on the phone as we look up at our moon. He enjoys this just as much as I do. This is our spiritual connection.

When I stopped and thought about these connections, I could see our level of love and support for one another, regardless of the difficult parts.

There has always been something about his hands that caught my eye from the very beginning. His hands were soft, tan, and beautiful. When I first touched his hand, I was surprised that his skin was smooth and felt like mine. I could feel the strength in him from his hands. It must be because my grandfather had those same hands, and they never let me down, so I equated the same to these new hands.

During our wedding ceremony, the person marrying us touched on how we can support one another in our marriage when she proclaimed, "These hands will be there..." while holding ours together in unity. Ever since we said "I do" and walked down the aisle hand in hand, swinging them in the air to celebrate us, I realized we had been there. When my grandmother died, John was by my side at the funeral, holding my hand. When his mother died, I was by his side, holding him up with my hands. When the time came to put our old dog to sleep, we both held him tight and reached for each other's hands. Reading the results of the pregnancy tests, he was there to put his arms around me. His hands wiped my tears. We have been there.

Back to our connection talk at the kitchen table, I finally was getting the answers I needed from him. I really wanted to understand what he felt if he didn't feel like failure.

"I admit I experienced jealousy watching friends and my brothers become fathers. I felt even empty at times," he told me.

"But did this make you feel less manly?" I wanted to know.

"No. Had nothing to do with that," he responded. This was interesting to me because his masculinity was not connected to these feelings of being without, like me.

I was surprised at his response when I asked him what the IVF treatment was like for him. He said, "More than anything, I was more concerned about you and the whole process. Yes, the masturbation room was weird, but I looked at it as just part of the process, what we had to do. I was more concerned about how you were dealing emotionally."

Huh. Here I was, resenting him for not feeling the same way as me when the hardest part for him was seeing me struggle emotionally.

"This was the reason I hated talking about it once we realized we were not going to be able to have children," he shared.

I thought he didn't care because he wouldn't talk about it, when really he was trying to protect me from the struggle by not talking about it. In his mind, if he could avoid the meltdown talks, he thought it was protecting me from having another one. But I needed those meltdowns to process the pain until I was done holding space for this.

I will never forget the country drive out to my wedding location. I wanted to drive that day in my old red Ford Explorer, and with my best friend in the passenger seat, we sang along to Led Zeppelin's "Ramble On." When we turned down the dirt road to the location site, there was an entire field full of the tallest and largest sunflowers I had ever seen. How had I not seen them before? I had been to the site several times before that day and never saw them. We were literally blown away by all of them. They were so impressive that the wedding guests stopped and took photos in the fields.

Sunflowers symbolize adoration, loyalty, and longevity. They are known for being the "happy" flowers, bringing joy to all they encounter. They lined the entire road to the ceremony site, smiling in the sun as if waving to us as we passed.

"I now present to you Mr. and Mrs. Weber," the wedding officiant announced.

I like the sounds of that. I smiled up at him as we turned toward our guests, the sun shining down on us; we squeezed our hands and walked back down the aisle together, toward the beginning of us.

Chapter 5

The Pressure Cooker

"The pressure of society we experience is caused by us. It can only dissipate when we stop pushing ourselves to live up to its standards."

JUN MAR PRADO

"Do you have children?"

Anyone I had a conversation with would ask. I learned I had to prepare what to say in response. I have changed my story a few times through the years. My initial response was, "Not yet," with an uncomfortable pause and my eyes lowered, "But we are trying." Even that would be hard to say without choking up.

I practiced saying this in the mirror with a smile, albeit forced. I would stand there proud, shoulders back, trying to look confident, shaking my hair, chin up.

I can do this. I let out a deep exhale and lowered my shoulders. *But I wish I didn't have to.*

"Not yet! But we are trying!" The look on my face, eyebrows lifted with a forced smile and a more-than-chipper voice, said it all.

Too fake.

Who is that cheerful? I mean, really, like, ever? I wanted to appear as if I was under control and not an emotional disaster. I didn't want anyone to see that part. Again. I looked into my eyes as if I was looking into whoever was asking me this. With a strong voice, with no cracking, firm in my affliction but light in tone, I said, "No, we don't have children, but we are trying. What about you?"

There, that felt better. My adult self could handle this, even though I did not care if they had children. That part was a lie.

Once I entered menopause and my periods stopped, I changed my response. This one had to come from my matter-of-fact tone with a quick staccato beat. "No, we do not have children. We tried for many years, and we were unable to have them." Exit stage left, drop the mic.

There, I said it.

I can now say this with absolute truth because it is. I looked in the mirror one last time, fluffed my hair up to boost the roots, checked in with my green eyes, then walked out and closed the bathroom door behind me.

Once I became aware of the impact of this hidden pressure, I learned to respond to the question differently. The reality is that people have no idea what I am going through, and I'm sure if they knew I was the infertile one in the room, they would not be asking me this question. In fact, they would feel terrible asking me this. It's like asking a blind person about the color of the sunset. By realizing the power this question had over my emotions, I was able to release the emotional trigger these words held over me. This shift in perspective was my first step outside the pressures of society. Stepping outside the box allowed me to open the door to observation.

To me, out of all the things that infertility brings, navigating how I fit into the mold of society's normal was the most challenging. On an emotional level, I felt I did not belong anywhere. The mold for women is this: you are expected to get married, and you are expected to have kids. That is it, and if you don't do one of those two things, then it feels as if the whole world is against you. This is a big idea to hold onto when it comes to feelings of isolation. When trying to survive infertility, the underlying pressure of society must be recognized and understood.

Often, my most significant revelations happened in the early morning hours. My mind was in a constant state of examination to process what was unraveling for me. At some point on the journey, I woke up before the sun rose, snuggled in my comfy bed with my husband still sleeping. *Why is this so hard?* I sat in this thought as my old dog Andy heard me stirring and jumped on the bed to be by my side. I scratched his belly and hugged him as I contemplated, eyebrows pinched as if trying to hear or see some magical writing on the wall. I thought if I squinted long enough, I might hear something; sometimes, I did. This particular morning, I heard this. *Society. Expectation. Culture norm. The world expects procreation from everyone.* Wow. That's it? I tilted my head on my pillow in contemplation. "That is it," I whispered out loud. When I became aware of this, I was then able to start to process and handle life situations more delicately. But until that moment of clarity was reached, there was no grace in those life moments.

When first meeting a new person, the cultural standard is to ask questions and get to know one another. Those questions look like this: where are you from, what do you do for work, are you married, and do you have kids? If the answer is no to the kids, the next question is, why? For me, during the heart of the struggle, I literally felt like punching the person in the face. I dreaded this question, and it happened daily, with what seemed like everyone, from strangers at a dinner party, on the plane, at a football game, on the street—I mean, everywhere all the time. I couldn't believe how many people would ask me this. Why do they care? What difference does it make? And that's when I began to realize this is a societal thing. Everybody is asking me because that is just what people are conditioned to do when first meeting. This is the universal script we were taught and what we expect in conversations. It is not meant to attack your well-being directly, but that is precisely what it feels like when the question is asked while suffering.

The pressure felt from the social implications of infertility is magnified in that the concept of family is literally the center of our social structure, guiding deep-rooted social norms that affect our behaviors.[4] It is the nature of our social standards to bear children and produce a family. What is not standard is to be barren, and it does not fit the social paradigm of the family that is expected. Conversations would end there because society does not have a dialogue designed to respond to infertility. It was uncomfortable to admit that we were having trouble getting pregnant because the conversation would just end there, magnifying inside that I was on the outside.

I don't fit in here.

The stress of infertility and the reminder of "without" can happen at any given moment. There I was, minding my own business, walking down Main Street of my hometown. It was a warm summer day with a slight breeze. The sidewalks were busy with foot traffic as people meandered in and out of storefronts. On the corner sat the town's well-known street musician, playing the blues on his electric guitar, looking a lot like ZZ Top's lead guitarist Billy Gibbons.

I stopped to cross the street, and there she was, a beautiful pregnant belly in a black sundress with a billowy straw hat. She was everything I wanted to be. I clenched my teeth, took a deep breath, and looked down as I passed by her. *You can't have this. You won't know this.* I fought to hold back the emotions and the tears that always follow. Then it's like children start falling out of the sky. Everywhere I looked, there they were of all ages: running with a balloon, eating a sucker, crying about nothing, and smiling about everything. *Not your life. You aren't in this one.* I have no choice but to cry softly behind my aviator sunglasses.

Many women of today are having children later in life, which is one reason why infertility is much higher than in the past. But still, the quest to bring forth life and evolve is very much ingrained in our DNA; it is our birthright. So, for those of us who don't have this, it is extremely painful to be asked that question and not know how to respond. The emotion that dwells in your stomach and then explodes out of your heart can trigger crocodile tears instantly. This is overwhelming. That is why I dreaded going anywhere where new people might be. I avoided moments like these at all costs.

One random day, I opened the mail to find a baby shower invitation. A close friend was having a baby. Another invite to another shower. *Can't wait.* I threw the invite down and stomped off to sit on the front steps outside with my dogs. The emotional weight of infertility brings forth a pain that feels never-ending. *Why is this pain so hard to get out from under?*

One of the first steps is becoming aware of our cultural norms. Bearing children is universal and expected of all of us. This is a massive idea for the entire planet, and when you look at it this way, it is easy to see how overwhelming not fitting into this ideal can feel. The norm revolves around the expectation to procreate as the reason we are here, which only adds immense pressure on the infertile ones who are unable to meet it.

With that, we all have to fit in somewhere as our minds naturally compartmentalize and compare. In this case, there are two groups: the fertile and the infertile. The fertile ones just think about getting pregnant, and it happens on the first try. One time for sex, first moon cycle, done. The infertile, well, this is the struggle into oblivion group—forty-two times, many moon cycles, nothing happening.

There was incredible shame experienced when I compared my life to what society says I should be. It was my self-inflicted measuring tool that I applied to my so-called model life. For me, what I was perceiving was that if I did not fit the criteria, then this was internalized and turned into self-defeating behavior. In these moments, the Void had the most power. The pain is high, life is not giving you what you want, and you cannot see a way out of it. You are dealing with a wide range of difficult emotions, and none feel good. Once shame is applied, a recipe for ultimate failure has now been created.

Here's what I learned. The pressures of society act as a spotlight on the pain of infertility. It contributed to the pain I was carrying around. When we experience pain, we just want it to go away. So, we look for ways to remove the situation or persons that are causing the pain. But you can't remove life. There is nowhere to hide from it. When I became aware of these pressures, I was able to learn to realign my energy outside of these societal expectations by honoring my life as it is. I would tell myself in my bathroom mirror, *You know what? You don't fit the mold, and there is no way you will naturally be able to. The sooner you can come to terms with this, the sooner we can start to move past the pain.* I was trying to shift my energy instead of aligning with these expectations. How can I align with something new that would allow me to identify with a higher vibration of thought, which would ultimately relieve the pressure?

ISOLATION

The desperation that comes from societal pressures is due to the isolation that comes with it. That is the root of the emotion. Who the hell wants to feel isolated? What a terrible feeling, no matter how old you are or what you are doing in life. It feels like shit because we are not connected. Connection is our natural way of being. However, when we are locked in pain, we are experiencing a hundred negative emotions of that pain. This is the most difficult part of the pain. It isn't defined by just one emotion. It is all of the bad ones at any given time. Maybe it would be more manageable if we only felt sad and not sad—versus sad plus angry then fucking pissed to raging to disappointed, to now I'm fat, I hate all people having babies, to jealousy to lesser than all beings to flat out depressed and my spirit crushed into a million little pieces. This is what infertility looks like in the mind. Living on these thoughts easily drives more reasons to dive deeper into isolation—the Void's ammo.

So I asked myself, *What is isolation? What am I doing to myself to feel this way?* In these moments of uncomfortableness, I was socially withdrawing from the situation (to escape the pain), which led me into social and emotional isolation. Socially withdrawing is avoiding people and activities you would usually enjoy. All types of social isolation can include staying home for lengthy periods, having no communication with family, acquaintances, or friends, and/or willfully avoiding any contact with other humans when those opportunities arise.

Emotional isolation is a state of isolation where one feels emotionally separated from others.[5] When we don't understand what we are feeling in our own skin, how can we share it with others? This happens when we have too many emotions happening at one time. It is confusing, so we shut it down in an effort to stop them from coming at us. It is like being swept away down a wild river, where the currents constantly shift and change, and you bump into rocks and logs, unclear of where you are going. Is this the beginning of going crazy? I stopped sharing my emotions and became emotionally isolated, floating alone on my little island. The danger of this is the negative effect it has on self-esteem. Isolation is more than separating yourself from your friends or difficult situations. Once disconnected emotionally, the world becomes a very dark place. Infertility brings out both social and emotional isolation.

When you are having a hard time, your support group wants to help, but they are at a loss for what to say. Because when you are engulfed in the state of mind of immense pain, you can't even hear them. This is the language of the Void and its purpose: to create separation from others and invite isolation into your reality.

I never knew about the Void until infertility. I had never felt alone, insecure, or deep sadness like this before. I was depleted of my natural state of being, which was comfortable, happy, and free. I was void of my connection with others. I was void of peace in my soul. The Void was so foreign to my existence, I knew that I had invited a dark entity of negative energy to take over me. I felt powerless because I could not change the way I was feeling, and I felt trapped in my own body because I could not see a way out of it. The Void changed the lens of my life to cloudy, dark, and sad. I knew this was not me. Ironic, because I invited the Void right in when I blocked my emotions to avoid the pain. This was to protect my heart and to feel nothing. *Here, I am safe.*

A few months after the failed IVF, I had a call that resulted in THE moment I blocked the pain and shut down. I wanted to try for another round of IVF, until that phone call with the doctor from the Seattle clinic.

"Mrs. Weber, this is Dr. Preston in Seattle," she announced. "In reviewing your records, I am sorry to say but you only have a one percent chance at success." She was short and to the point. I was silent and in disbelief.

"I am sorry, can you tell me that again? Are you saying we have no chance?" I managed to respond.

"Correct. I would not recommend moving forward with another IVF treatment. Your chances are very low and highly unlikely for a positive outcome."

"I guess we won't be having another treatment then." I stood in my living room in shock. *This really is the end. This is not happening.*

Once I understood that isolation is the state of the mind created by the emotions generated from the pain, I could stop the Void from coming in and creating that division. The Void loves the separation and wants to keep us alone and not connected. What fun is that? When we are at our lowest, that is when we need others the most to help us through. Connection with our peers is so important to get support. I could not get love by hiding and isolating myself. I was perceiving my world as separate, and that is exactly what I was presenting to others. I was showing that I wanted to be left alone, and so that is what happened. Now, I have created a world blocked out, and not only does that feel terrible, but dangerous to my overall well-being.

For me, while in the throws of the battle, I did not speak openly of my hardship. But I did talk with my husband, my mother, my best friend, and my sister-in-law. That was my core support group. However, in the darkest hour I began to hide my feelings, even to them. I preferred to drink wine alone and listen to depressing music from Coldplay. I would drink too much, cry, and dance around my living room in sorrow. Okay, maybe I was stumbling around searching for answers in my stupor, but it felt like dancing at the time. Back in the bathroom, I would sway in front of the mirror and work to focus on my sad face. "God, you look terrible," I would share with myself. And I did. My face was gray with sadness. I have a great smile and a big mouth, and when I'm happy, I often laugh with a great, deep, guttural laugh. Nothing feels better than the shake of the whole body in laughter. Even better, the shit-eating grin that follows.

But in these moments, this laughter and smile were nowhere in sight. I had a permanent bitch face. Staring in the mirror, I would make terrible attempts at a smile, resulting in my upper lip half curled to the side, like a dog with his upper lip caught on his canine teeth. "Great, I can't even smile anymore." I slammed my hands down against the light switch, marched to my bedroom, and fell backward into the bed with my arms stretched out. *Someone catch me.*

I learned that avoiding life forever wasn't going to work for me. This is important to recognize. But while you are in a great time of pain, give yourself a break and know it is okay to skip some of the hard parts, like baby showers. Baby showers are the single most difficult event to attend when suffering. And they are everywhere because everyone you know is having a baby. Not only that, but there are usually three or four other pregnant women there too. It's like baby life on steroids. And for those of you in the struggle, oh my goodness, look out. You are walking into the greatest pain-trigger moment of them all.

I attended my fair share of them until the last one put me over the edge. There was country music playing in the background. I was wearing a white sundress with little yellow flowers and a blue jean jacket. You know, a baby shower-type wardrobe, which I chose to appear happy. The living room was packed, so I sat on the outskirts of the scene on the wool carpet, leaning against the heavy leather furniture. Surrounded by pregnant women, we watched the Mommy-to-be open gifts. All I could think was, *I want this to be me right now.* Oh shit. This belief has now invited the Void to the party. I was already hiding in full panic, so these thoughts came down on me hard. Much worse, they were armed with a gas can. Let the dumpster fire begin.

I really couldn't hear what anyone else was saying in the room as they ogled over the little baby clothes held up in the air. My vision began to narrow, and I felt light-headed. *Am I going to pass out right now?* The tears were literally right under the surface, about to explode. I needed to escape and thought about making a run for it right out the front door, saying nothing to anyone as I left. I had visions of myself running and crying all the way down the street. Talk about fight-or-flight syndrome. I let out four deep breaths as I held on strong to my fake smile. I had no choice but to fight my way through this uncomfortable moment. I could feel heat rising up and into the back of my neck. Tiny beads of sweat were forming on my forehead. While most people in that room knew we were trying, they had no idea the pain I was suffering internally. I was hanging on for dear life. I imagined myself freaking out and standing up in the middle of the room, kicking the baby gifts, screaming, "I HATE BABY SHOWERS."

Sitting there listening to these doomed thoughts of panic, I couldn't take it anymore. I got up and went to the restroom and cried my eyes out. Great. Now I've got red, puffy eyes at a baby shower—my worst nightmare. I grabbed a washcloth and ran cold water on it in an effort to cheer up my eyeballs. I exhaled and stared at myself in the mirror, and that's when I knew this would be the last baby shower I would ever attend. I distinctly remember the navy blue wallpaper with wildflowers in that bathroom and the curved curtain rod. Wallpaper. Who has wallpaper? I was searching for something to switch my focus to so I could get out of the panic. I just couldn't bear the pain in a public setting. A pain this great is not meant to be shared at a baby shower. This shower was not about me; it was about my friend celebrating the life that was joining her family. I went back out, grabbed a glass of wine, and put my fake smile back on. It took all the courage in the world to finish that baby shower.

Now, I had read that not attending baby showers for a while was okay if the pain was too great to attend. That line saved me. I learned to be honest with myself and with my friends and family. They were very supportive and understood, and boy, did this bring me a sense of relief. In fact, my business partner once invited me like this: "I know you don't want to go to any of these, but I wanted to include you anyway. I totally understand if you cannot be there." This was the best thing anyone had ever said to me. This gave me permission to bow out. "Thank you. I will be there in spirit." And that was that.

What I regret is not sending a baby gift to them. I just could not do it. I couldn't even walk down baby aisles at Target without crying. I would walk down the baby aisle at grocery stores like a funeral procession, slowly looking at the pacifiers, the tiny toenail clippers, diapers, and baby wipes and pushing my cart in silence as I held my breath. *I will never need to buy these.* Then, I would go to the wine aisle and buy wine.

The first Christmas with all the new nephews together was a tough one. My husband's family came to town, his two brothers and their little babies everywhere. I kept it together by being busy making Christmas special with holiday cookies and hot chocolate drinks. I wasn't too worried about it until suddenly, on the Eve of Christmas, we sat in the living room around the tree with the fireplace roaring in the background. We watched the children pick out one present to open from under the tree. Everyone was swooning over the growth of the family in the way life delivered those sweet messages of love. It was a rite of passage moment for the grandparents as they watched their boys become fathers and start traditions with their own.

But one of their boys did not have a child. John didn't seem as affected by this scene. We never talked about it. But for me, these words repeated in my head. *You are not a part of this moment. You don't have children.* I could feel the Void grow stronger. The sadness was stirred and was beginning to take over. At least I was in my own house this time. The tears were filling up fast, and then my body began to shake as I held my grief tight to my chest. I put on my best fake smile again, then retreated to my bathroom floor for a good hour's cry.

Another year while decorating the tree, I thought, "Maybe this time next year, there will be a little baby sleeping in the room while I decorate this tree." I wished for that as I placed the gold star on top of the tree. I imagined the ornaments I would hang in honor of our new baby and family. That made me smile and dream of that special moment. But the next year came, and the next one after that, and decorating the tree became a reminder of a dream that would never come true.

As life kept presenting these moments to me, I continued my quest of how to survive these times without meltdowns. I questioned often, *will this ever end?* I started by trying hard to fit into what society said to do. I even decorated our front door for Halloween. Until one day, I stopped that too. We don't have kids; who am I decorating for, my forty-five-year-old husband? That is the reason I have never sent Christmas cards, either. It was part of my retaliation toward life. I'm not sending cards, and I'm not decorating for Halloween, period.

I knew in my heart I could not continue down this path and avoid life forever. I needed connection to survive. While society's expectations will continue to evolve, one thing I knew would never change was everyone's desire to procreate. This would always be a factor, so I had to learn to let go of that. It is not going anywhere. One good thing that has shifted in society is there is more acceptance of couples without children. Younger generations are not as focused on having children as we were. They want to establish their lives and careers first and spend time with their partners before becoming parents, if they ever decide to be parents. Through these connections, I felt more like the old me, and then it slowly started to happen: the intense energy of the pressure began to lift.

Here are a few key elements I found to help alleviate the pressure.

1. Accept the possibility that your life is just as it should be. One of my favorite sayings was and is, "It is what it is." This saying got me through the toughest moments. I said this out loud when I hung up with the IVF doctor who told me to call it quits. There was nothing more to say than *it is what it is.* By saying this out loud, I was able to accept what was happening to me and keep any emotional outbreaks at bay.

2. Honor the pain. Our lives are filled with lessons so we can learn about ourselves. We can never escape the painful ones; these are the most powerful ones. To survive the difficult moments in the lesson, instead of avoiding the painful parts, I began to allow the experience to unfold, giving myself permission to feel

through the hard stuff. Here, I was holding space for the pain to do its work.

3. Acknowledge the hard emotions, and don't fight to keep them out. I would greet each emotion as it showed up. *Oh, hello, anger and rage, there you are. What do you got for me today? Let's go.* Granted, I might have been a little pissed off at my hard emotions, but meeting them at the door took a little wind out of their sails in their sneaky self-destructive ways.

When I focused on accepting, honoring, and acknowledging my pain, this made the pressure of it all a little easier. Soon, baby showers were just baby showers, and holidays could pass by with ease.

Ultimately, the pressure I was feeling was coming from within. No one was putting this on me, but me. It was all me, pushing myself to live up to these standards of society. *Why can't I have my own standards?* When I began to push back on society standards and not accept them as mine, my pressure released. Besides, it is too stressful to carry the weight of the world around all day. And you know what's great about that? We don't have to.

Chapter 6

What Not to Do

"The only thing more exhausting than being depressed is pretending that you're not."

ANONYMOUS

I was officially depressed. While there are a million things we should not do when we are in a depressed state, these are the ones that, in the long run, hurt me the most: trying to escape my feelings with booze, comparing myself with the fertile people, and designing the nursery. All of these decisions provided zero support to my nervous system and overall well-being. Instead, these only added fuel to the fire when I needed water and a life vest the most.

BOOZE CONTROL

I'll never forget the summer of Budweiser. After my third miscarriage (the one where I actually got a heartbeat), I decided I would drink as much Budweiser as possible. Fuck it. You could say this was not one of my brighter moments in life. It's one thing to drink for fun, at social events, or while golfing or enjoying a dinner with friends, versus drinking as many Budweisers as possible, pretty much every day, and, at the very worst, alone. If you have an underlying tone of fuck it, I don't care, I'm pissed, who gives a shit anyway, then you have got a problem. That was me in the summer of Budweiser. Instead of keeping my hormones at bay, I looked toward booze control to keep my pain and suffering at bay.

I won't lie. It is very easy to pick up a bottle when you are depressed and sad. It does numb the pain for a little bit. It makes you feel normal in the social world for a little bit. You stop thinking about your problems for a little bit. This is why I consciously made the choice to drink. This was the only way I knew how to let go in that moment. I put the intention into it just in the words *fuck it*, which I thought every time I opened another Bud.

In my case, the summer of Budweiser was purposely driven to not give a shit. It should have been my red flag. My choice to get on booze control to handle the stress got me nowhere but deeper into the spiral of discontent.

We lived in a tiny two-bedroom rental downtown. I was sitting on the back porch in a faded lawn chair at sunset one early summer evening. I cracked open a Budweiser and sat there alone, crying and crying and crying. There was a gentle breeze, just enough to push the smell of the lilac bushes through the air. The more I drank, the fuzzier my brain got, and the more my mental game escaped me. I was powerless in those moments. No clarity to stop my negative mind, literally drinking my sorrows away. All I had for comfort was the occasional aroma of the lilacs.

Lucky for me, my phone rang, and I answered, dumping all of my tears on my friend, filled with rambling words of nonsense. She listened in silence until I finally ran out of words to say, "Well, then buck up and get over the fact you are having a hard time getting pregnant." Um, that didn't go over well, as it ignited a huge meltdown. I hung up and started yelling our conversation out loud to myself. "SHE SAYS JUST FUCKING GET OVER IT. REALLY? REALLY, DID SHE JUST FUCKING SAY THAT TO ME?" *Good God, can the neighbors hear me freaking out over here?* I imagined someone yelling over the fence, "YAH, SHE DID SAY THAT TO YOU. SHUT THE FUCK UP." I rolled out and off the lawn chair, kicked it and shoved it off the deck, and stomped my way back into the house.

I was in such dire straits, and the only logical thing to do in that moment was to put on my wedding dress. This was the last day of my life that I could remember being happy. Maybe if I put the dress on, I can get some of that happy back. The windows were open, the white curtains were lightly swaying in the breeze, and the smell of lilacs moved through the room with ease. While the reality was serene, the emotions were raging and thrashing inside. I was so drunk that I got the zipper caught and ruined the dress. The dress had a mesh overlay and got tangled in the zipper. I could barely get the damn thing off. Then I was super pissed, staggering around the house with the wedding dress half on, and this triggered a crying fit on the wood floor surrounded by mesh. I laid back and stared at the popcorn ceiling as the sweet smell of lilacs surrounded me once again. Maybe this is what finally stopped the tantrum. Now my dress is ruined forever. I still don't have kids. But I have a huge hangover to look forward to instead. *Winning.*

This moment pops into my head every time I open the closet that stores my wedding dress. I think of this day instead of the memory of my wedding day and how beautiful that moment in time was to me. For a long time afterward, I would stand there, sigh, and slam the door. There it is again, a little reminder of pain.

In the toughest times, I found that I was spending my energy either running away, masking the pain, or drowning in sorrow underneath my wedding dress. That's what alcohol does for us. It is only a vice to try and get away from it all. What were the words in my mind as I drank the night away? *I'll show you.* When I think about that now, show who? Who was I talking to? I was so angry that infertility was happening to me. I was angry at everyone. My husband, my family, and my friends, no one knew what to say to me. Infertility defined my emotions in that part of my life, and I hated it. I could not flip a switch to turn it off. This was my life, and it felt like shit all day and all night. The pain would not stop, and it was always there waiting for me. I was only witnessing my own demise.

Now I tell people about the summer of Budweiser and how I thought getting on booze control was a good idea. I never mention raising my Bud in the air as I sat in my lawn chair nightly, secretly saying "fuck you" to pregnancy, per can. Instead, I say it was fun (well, some of the time). Nevermind the fact that I got as fat as shit drinking Bud heavies.

I also omit the fights and the meltdowns alcohol would ignite between my husband and me. The need to talk about my emotions always felt more comfortable after a bottle of wine, but look out; I was out of control once the mascara was smeared. My husband would be like, "Oh no, here we go. She's going to go crazy on me." He looked frightened while trying to shut me down. This would infuriate me. *HOW CAN HE NOT WANT TO TALK ABOUT THIS WITH ME?* (said the insane woman shooting fire out of her eyes). But when you are drunk, you can't see that he was running for his life while trying to stop the meltdown-freak-out cry fight before it happened. That was his worst nightmare. And it happened over and over and over again. Half the time, I couldn't remember what mean thing I had just said right after saying it, and then he would walk out. There I would be, crying on the floor (my favorite place to be), and it felt like shit. I would wake up in the morning, apologize, and feel even worse.

Alcohol serves only as a distraction. The irony is that drinking to calm the sadness of infertility is the last thing I should have turned to for my mind and the worst thing for my body. Alcohol is a depressant. It affects the mind and body in so many negative ways if abused. It brings cloudiness to your brain, and decisions are often terrible while under the influence.

What I learned is that booze control was not the answer. It blurred my heart, mind, and soul connection and damn near ruined my marriage. It lowered my vibration and made me feel terrible overall. It disrupted the connection with my spirit. Booze control became my silent story of drinking my sorrows away; I was drinking myself away. Yes, it feels good to be numb; that's why I did it. At that moment, the escape was worth it. But by the end of the night, I knew the Void was waiting patiently to attack my broken heart.

COMPARISON TO THE FERTILE ONES

I was sitting in the terminal waiting to board our flight. It was early in the morning. A sliver of sunrise peaked from behind the mountains, and a mom with her two children walked up to the Delta gate. One was about three years old and on foot, the other the age of one, in a stroller that looked to be a nightmare to fold up. I watched as the younger one drank milk with sleepy eyes, relaxing contentedly in her seat, while the other one took off toward the next gate and then the next as he gained speed. You could see the mom was tired, maybe because of the early morning hours or simply the balancing act needed to maintain a household with one- and three-year-olds. She ran after him in a flash and grabbed his right arm, half dragging him back to where she had left the stroller. Me, I sipped on my coffee and watched this all play out. What does she feel like right now? After she managed to talk the three-year-old into standing in one place for a hot second (I think she squeezed his collarbone a little), she pulled down her Athleta jacket, took a sip of coffee, and let her shoulders relax. Was she thinking,

"Damn. I love this motherhood shit. I'm a goddamn rock star"? Or, "How in the hell am I going to make it all the way to Atlanta with these two? I hope they don't scream on the airplane." While I'll never know how she felt at that moment, I did know that she had it all.

When you are infertile, it is easy to compare yourself to those who are not. I was so trapped in my bubble of hell that I was living my life (other than the booze) as if I had children. We were not jet-setting across the globe, sipping margaritas on the beaches of luxurious boutique hotels, playing golf wherever we wanted, hiking through the Amazon, diving in Belize, visiting temples in Thailand, or drinking our way through Italy. Instead, we were working at the office, then coming home. That was it. My time was filled with scouring the internet, searching for new leads on how to conceive fast, what was the next approach, when, where, and how much. We were living month-to-month off of my cycle. We were so focused on trying to conceive that nothing else really mattered. Nothing else was in focus.

The mothers I knew complained about sleep deprivation, as well as struggling to get their child to eat, pee in a toilet, take a nap, and sleep through the night while fighting with the notion of the change in independence that often strikes motherhood in the beginning. I found a commonality, although odd, in my silent comparisons. There was a comfort in knowing that they, too, struggled. While our struggles were complete opposites of the spectrum, this comfort was my only connection to motherhood, to sisterhood. But the reality is, and was, there is no comparison. Those mothers would never want to walk in my shoes. The experience of the childless woman is not the same.

I sort of let life pass by for a while when we should have been out there living—traveling everywhere, meeting new people, learning new things, whatever I wanted, because I had the time and the freedom. I remember going to Nebraska football games and watching intently as mothers wrangled their kids through the gates to their seats and ensured they had everything they needed. Even in those moments, I would feel the sorrow of not having that because I was comparing. I finally realized I had to stop comparing my life to the fertile people. All I could see in the comparison was that one heart was full and the other, mine, was empty. While both experiences are equally hard and can have moments of emotional drain, in the end the two lives cannot be measured. I had to let that go.

Here's the thing: it's natural to compare your life to others, especially on this topic. If you believe the fertile ones have it all and you don't, you are walking right into the depression of it all. It's like opening the door to your heart to give the sadness of the Void room to grow. So how do we stop this automatic comparison that seems to happen without our permission?

Much of my realizations happened through ideas planted after deep contemplation. I would often find myself staring into space—on my couch, on my front porch, as soon as I woke up, in my car, drinking coffee, laying in the grass, in between work calls, washing dishes, getting gas, walking down a golf course, hiking in the mountains, taking a shower, waiting in any line. Here, in these simple life moments, I examined my emotions, my world, and my experience in hopes of finding a way out of the pain I lived in. One day, it dawned on me. *You are not on the same path as your mother friends.* With this message, I began to see a new way to connect again with the fertile ones. Even though I was not on the motherhood path, focusing my energy on asking about the phases of raising children—are they sleeping through the night, eating soft foods, potty training, enjoying T-ball practice— was all I had to do to be included in the conversations. Because this was all that fertile ones were thinking about. My personal path was not this. I did not need to think about any of these things. I was headed down a path of self-discovery through pain and suffering. A much different experience than the life of a mother. So, I found it easy to engage and ask the obvious questions that all mothers were living.

"How is potty training going?"

Ask any question about child rearing, and the fertile ones will gladly discuss what is happening in their world. While this was difficult for me at first, the more I pushed myself to ask the questions, the more at ease I was able to stay in the conversation. At first I did not care about the answers and faked my way through it. It was hard to put myself in those conversations. But once I got out of my own way, I was able to become more supportive of their trials and tribulations as parents. It was my hope that they could understand my life without children, although no one wanted to deep dive into that part. Today, I look at my life as unique and that I am here to experience a much different life than those with children. I came to know this much through many moons of silent contemplation without comparison.

THE NURSERY

I thought of it the day I decided to try and get pregnant. My business partner, who had an infant at the time, said to me, "Are you sure you should be planning a nursery already?" Maybe that is what jinxed me right out of the gate. I remember pausing at that statement but was like, "Yes, why wouldn't I?" I had picked out the warm room in my house, as the other one was ice cold, and I didn't want my baby freezing all the time. The room was on the northeast corner of the house and full of light with two big windows. I had imagined where the crib would go, the changing table, and the white puffy armchair where I would spend my time nursing and rocking my baby to sleep.

I would decorate everything with owls. I was going to wait to find out if a boy or girl, and owls would work with both. I would have pinks and greens and blues. I had already started looking online for baby sheet sets and cute sayings to hang on the wall. There was everything owl out there, from lamps to pillows to little owl mobiles. I wanted it all. Dreaming of my nursery made me so happy and excited for what would come.

Three long years later, that nursery dream began to fade. I kept going into the designated room and then would cry. *Will I ever get my nursery in here?* I never actually bought anything for the nursery, partly because I listened to my business partner, and mostly because nothing was happening. But I could still dream and think about it. I would sit in there and imagine folding the baby clothes, and how cute my baby would be wearing all of them. I could see myself in the early morning hours, sitting in the white puffy chair, looking out the window as my baby slept in my arms. I could feel this moment in my bones.

In a way, this was me in mourning. There was no baby. There was no nursery—only me and the not-as-cold room in my house. When I learned that I had a one percent chance to conceive if I tried IVF again, that and the combination of my periods drying up, I realized that all that was left was to focus on myself. This was when I realized I was done crying in this room—and if I couldn't have a child, I would make this almost-nursery into something just for me. This room would become my safe haven, sanctuary, and sacred space. This room would later become my meditation room.

I still needed it for a guest room, so I worked around that and created my space. I hung soft white curtains. I built a platform bed and lined it with off-white sheets with a tribal dark blue and white duvet cover. I added all my plants, crystals, and Buddha statues and finished it by hanging my newfound totem animal, the gray-horned owl, who represents courage. This was my first step to healing from the pain of infertility. I needed this. I needed this space not to be about having a baby. How ironic that the very room where I chose to sit and mourn my unborn child for many years is now my sacred space. I meditate daily here, and now I create and write my stories in here. What a meaningful space this has become to me.

Mourning is part of the process of letting go. It is perfectly normal to dream about the nursery before having children; it is part of the process. Can you imagine if I had designed the room like "if you build it, they would come"? What an emotional disaster it would be to walk into an empty nursery only to resonate with the failure of conceiving. I'm surprised I did not create the nursery, as I am such a planner with little to no patience. The point is, when letting go of the pain that has a hold of you, look for things that bring you pleasure and peace to fill its place. For me, that was creating a space to invite peace and calm into my heart. I knew that if I had this room, I could retreat to it anytime to rest within my solitude, meditate, and write to my heart's desire.

Today, I don't even think about my sacred space as the old nursery room. Those thoughts are far from my mind. This room has seen everything out of me, down to the depths of my soul in the hardest of my emotional breakdowns, raw in my anger and grief. As I mourned, these four walls held me as I cried on the floor. Today, they uplift me for the woman I have become. It is my healing space where I go to find comfort and clarity. My salt lamp is always on, my meditation pillow waits patiently for me, the singing bowl rests in the corner of the room, and my plants send me loving energy as the crystals shine their high vibrations on me. This is now my safe space, my happy place.

We all cope in different ways. You might find you relate to some of my choices, or none at all. I invite you to identify your very own "what-not-to-dos." Once you discover those choices, then do and be the opposite. Make it positive and something that will bring comfort to your overall well-being.

Chapter 7

Get My Mind Right

"Life is ten percent of what happens to you and ninety percent how you react to what happens to you. And so it is with you...we are in charge of our attitudes."

CHARLES R. SWINDOLL

LOOPS AND EGOS

It was a lazy summer Sunday, a few months after hearing that we had a one percent chance to conceive if we tried IVF again. My husband and I went for a three-hour paddleboard float on the Madison River. I strapped the bright orange life jackets on my two border collies and gently pushed my board into the water as I sat down on it and paddled away from the river's edge. Even though the idea is to stand up on the paddle board to ride the water, I often sit down with my legs crossed and paddle, much like I am on a small raft. It is the most relaxing, laying on my back and letting the water take me where it wants to go. That day, as I lay back on my board, I looked up at the clouds. I could hear the ripple of the water flow beneath me. My dogs were splashing close by, swimming between John and me as we made our way down the river. At this moment, I was relaxed and able to feel a sense of peace.

Oh shit, this isn't going to work out as you planned.

Wait, what? I questioned my random thought out of nowhere. Seriously? This voice was relentless in its negative message, each word dripped with sarcasm, like an annoying neighbor or stepsister, or much like the fictional character "Karen" who the world has labeled as the living worst.

Yeaaaaaah, this is a major problem, a huge disappointment.

As I listened, the words only got worse.

We are not going to succeed. Failure is everywhere. The life plan is over.

And so it began—the chatter that would drive my daily thoughts, and consume my mind with negative beliefs that only served to fuel my mental suffering. This is the voice of the Void, and when repeated, the language of the Void becomes "the loops." The power of the loops comes from the brain's tendency to believe something the more it is repeated. The loops kept me on a negative belief track, on repeat, over and over again, looping and looping, and ultimately shaping my mindset and outlook on life.

While deep in the experience of infertility, my mind was uncomfortable, anxious, and confused. I wish I could say I was able to grasp what was happening to me. That my mind remained calm and centered while guiding me through the turbulent terrain of my emotions. This, it was not. My mind was unstable, and I had accepted to live in panic mode because nothing else was working. I was so consumed with the pain that I succumbed to it. There were no positive thoughts to be had. No matter how hard I tried to find them, to find something that made me smile, it was not there. All of my energy was tuned into panic. It was so powerful to me and a constant feeling during this time that I began to think it was normal. I simply did not know how to un-panic myself. On the outside, my face was furrowed in concern. On the inside, my guts were twisted and churning in distraught. My heart rate was rampant and erratic. In my mind, and at any given moment, thoughts of devastation would appear out of thin air, like that day on the river.

What I soon realized was that I was stuck in panic mode. I could not get out of these distraught thoughts. As I daydreamed about decorating the nursery, folding tiny baby clothes, and wearing fun maternity outfits, instead of feeling joy, I felt sheer panic that I might never get to experience any of it.

Lying under the glaze of panic was the deep remorse and mourning for the life of motherhood never lived. What I didn't know at the time was how good the mind was at keeping me in the trap. My brain developed layers of loops that were wired specifically for the pain, to keep me there as long as possible to help me survive by focusing on the threat. It's as if my brain was a record skipping, stuck on words that held me tighter in the center of pain, creating a never-ending trap. In processing the reality of a womb with no life, any expectations I had of my life were crushed and replaced with this monster mind of fear.

I first became aware of the Void from the healing with Carl, which took place three years into trying to get pregnant. The Void was the perfect name for my generalized anxiety disorder, mostly because the Void symbolized my separation from my peace and core belief systems. It took me another five years to understand that there were three phases to the Void in how it works to get a hold of your mind.

First there is a hook, then a loop, which in turn creates the trap.

1. The hook starts with a trigger thought like before. *Oh shit, this isn't going to work out as you planned.* It is what you do next that determines how this hook will play out. Will the hook turn into a loop or fade away?
2. Thoughts come and go through our minds. Some of them we let pass by, but some grab our attention, and when we follow them, usually another one like it will come next. When we follow, we attach belief to the idea. If we follow the hook, then this opens

the door to the loops. The longer my mind entertained these loops, the fear woven into these loops started to feel more and more like truth to me.

3. The loop's job is to fuel the trap created by the mind, and this is where the Void wants us. The trap keeps us stuck inside the core of the problem, with no way to see out. It is here we find the source of the pain, our very own mind telling us what to think and feel about the problem.

Once the loops feel like truth, then the trap has been set. This is where we get stuck, unaware, and miserable in our own minds. Our reality is a reflection of our thoughts, and yet, it is our minds that have the power to break free from it in a remarkable twist of fate. We have the ability to steer our minds in a positive direction, to get the mind right, but sometimes it takes listening to the spirit of our heart to help us get there. It feels like a kind of grace that helps us find a way out of the loops. Here, we can detach from the trap.

The brilliance of the mind is that it is so damn good at sneaking the loops in on us that we don't even see what is happening. Our focus is on dealing with the pain, right? How do we fix this? How do we get out of this? How can we survive? Meanwhile, the loops are playing in the background, keeping us trapped in the center of the heartache. *You are never going to get your dream.* What I found myself doing in these moments is trying to think my way out of the problem. While sometimes the negative thought pattern can serve as a protection, *I need to watch out when I walk down this dark alley,* it is when these thoughts become excessive that the mind gets caught working against us.

With my mind functioning in this way, stuck in the loops, the trap would leave me feeling perplexed, off, and lost. I knew no other way but to try and rationalize my way out of it. *When will this stop? Why do I feel this way? I can't have a baby. Medical intervention says no. So why are we still sitting in this mess? Why can't I move on? Why?* I really don't know how many months went by as I asked these questions because this time period feels like a blur. If I had to guess, I would say around six months of asking this question after I knew my body was not going to produce. The final IVF call really put the nail in the coffin.

I had an awareness through one of my morning meditations, like a knowing as I focused on my breathing. *Wow, your breathing is fucked up.* Okay, well, I didn't say it was an earth-shattering moment, but it did shift my thinking to my body. After that, I began to tune into my body more. How was it feeling? What I found was a rapid heartbeat along with shifts in my breathing at random times throughout the day. Mostly, I found myself holding my breath, yet nothing was consistent. All that was clear was that it didn't feel good, and my analytical mind wanted to understand why. A big part of it was I was resting in a constant state of fear, and when you sit in fear, your body is going to respond to it.

My a-ha moment was this: If I can figure out how to calm my body, then I can get out of this. When I had this thought, I turned my attention again to the why. Why does my body feel this way? What I figured out is what you tell yourself drives the body's sensations. It responds! If I can change the way I am thinking about this, I can change the way I feel, and if I can do that, then I can get out of my personal hell (that I created) and be free from this pain.[6]

Thank God for the internet. I scoured through websites and articles to try and identify what was happening to my body. What resonated most with me was the fight-or-flight response. It was showing up to match my stress, a physiological reaction that occurs in the presence of something that is terrifying, either mentally or physically, real or not. The fight-or-flight response releases hormones that prepare the body to either stay and deal with the threat or to run away to safety. The purpose of this response, and why we need it, is so that we can better perform under pressure and survive. Gauging from the way my body was responding to the stress, I was definitely working within this fight-or-flight energy.

American physiologist Walter Cannon discovered this engrained survival instinct after discovering how the body prepares and reacts to manage threatening situations. Through the years, psychologists have refined this response and developed two more responses known as freeze and fawn.

These responses are as follows:

1. Fight - confronting perceived threats aggressively
2. Flight - escaping or running away from danger.
3. Freeze - being immobilized or unable to act in the face of a threat.
4. Fawn - seeking to please or appease in order to avoid danger or conflict.[7]

I danced between all but fawn, but mostly I hung out in the fight zone, grinding teeth, glaring at everything, resisting the urge to kick and scream and even punch someone. Pretty much like a wild animal. It was only when I was in the trap, in the panic, that I froze. Learning about the hormones involved in the fight response, adrenaline and cortisol, and understanding that progesterone is needed to support them, all I could think of was my stolen progesterone being depleted on the fight response, when I needed it most to conceive!

So, how does this actually help me with infertility stress? The moment I learned that my body was programmed to cope by using the fight-or-flight response, everything changed. My body's reaction was happening whether I wanted it to or not, and I could not control it. What I could do was try to understand it, to recognize the symptoms my body was showing me, to become aware of why I was feeling these reactions like rapid heartbeats, clenched jaw, stomach aches, headaches, pressure on my chest, etc. The more I tuned into what my body was telling me, I soon realized the fight-or-flight response was not always accurate. While the thought of failing to become a mother and creating a family is terrifying, it is not life or death. To me, the fight-or-flight response is not needed to cope with this particular situation. But the loops were feeding the fight-or-flight response and keeping me in it. My body did not know the difference. For all my body knew, I could have been running for my life from jaguars in the jungle.

When I switched my focus from my loops to how my body was feeling, I brought awareness to the sensations of my body in response to the stress. This is important because your body is a tool of communication, and if we listen here first, then we have a chance to stop the loops before they start. Oftentimes, I did not pay attention to how I was physically feeling because I was trapped in the loop. It does not feel good when your heart is racing, and your breath is uneven. I was constantly grabbing my chest and taking deep breaths to control my breathing and rapid heartbeat, while my thoughts continued running rampant, driving the fear deeper into my shaky body. This is what panic feels like. Becoming aware of what my body was doing flushed me out of my mind, and I eventually stopped the attack. My focus shifted to calming the body. The loops were not going to help here as they were only interested in creating more agitation for the body.

Why is it so easy to get trapped and follow these loops down the rabbit hole of emotional disaster? I was on a mission to find out more. Curled up on my couch, with my dog lying next to me, I opened my computer and typed in the word "panic." Thanks to Google, I came across an article from *Psychology Today* and discovered that the loops have a medical name called rumination. When we are ruminating, we are repetitively going over a thought or a problem without completion. According to *Psychology Today*, common themes of rumination include thoughts of inadequacies and worthlessness when we are experiencing depression. These thought patterns raise the anxiety level, which creates more stress and brings a number of stress hormones into play. When this happens, the clarity to problem solve is challenged. With these ruminating thoughts, emotion attaches, which feeds our heartbroken pain, and then we continue to analyze how to stop the pain we are feeling.[8]

THIS was monumental for me. THIS is what was happening to me. THIS made sense. I felt a sense of relief now that I knew how my mind and body were reacting to infertility. *I am not staying here.* Now that I knew, I could find a way out. Sometimes, when reading an article, blog, or book that speaks to you as if written for you, to you—when you find these words that your whole being resonates with—it is like a gift from your angels. Like hearing a song on the radio with the exact message you needed at that moment. That is what I experienced when Google brought this article to me. It was that kind of moment.

Unfortunately for me, this new awareness did not stop the loops immediately. My brain still needed time to process the problem. *Great. Patience is not my thing.* The biggest part of that is that what I wanted, my greatest desires, were not happening in my life. Because of this, my brain focused on the why and how to take action to go get it for me. Amazing how the brain is designed to function this way, to align you with your desires. Whether or not the alignment was in my cards was another thing. Here are what my infertility loops sounded like:

What if it never happens to me?

I have nothing to share in parenting conversations.

Outsider for life.

Something is wrong with you.

I'm never going to know what it is like to have a baby.

Who will take care of us when we are older?

What did we do wrong, God?

When will this pain go away?

I will never be pregnant.

I will never have a baby shower.
I will never be called Mommy.
We will never have a first Christmas.
Will I ever be okay again?
Will I ever feel whole again?
Why didn't God pick us?
I will never know unconditional love.
I will never know the mother-child relationship.
I will never be a woman.

Some of these loop themes stayed with me for several weeks at a time. They may have even played out on the same day as my mind rolled through each and every one of them and, even worse, believed them. Overall though, I was trapped in these loops for years. Once I became aware that my mind was on repeat with thoughts leading me nowhere, I knew I had to figure out a way to get out of them. I no longer wanted to identify with this thought pattern. Mindfulness was the answer. Living mindlessly intensifies the pain because the mind left unattended has a negative mindset. When I became aware of the loops as they happened and began to observe rather than believe, over time I was able to stop myself from getting caught within the landscape of the trap.

Then I questioned my ego: *why can't you just be on my side for once?* Our thoughts carry the energy of negative or positive. The ego is the one creating the thoughts based on how it perceives reality. If the ego is hurt, it will generate negative thoughts, and then we feel the conflict in the body, and our body actually aches physically.[9] I felt this like a dagger in my heart, twisting. If I could let go of the ego (the part of me feeling and perceiving the pain), then maybe the grip of that pain would start to loosen, if not recede entirely. When it comes to conceiving, ironically we are faced with the outcome of either a positive or a negative, and the emotions that are tied to these results carry the energy of positive or negative thoughts. Literally, when you want to conceive and you get the positive on the pee stick, the elated feeling of success and the emotions of joy attached to this positive sign instantaneously remove the pain of infertility. It's like, poof, the pain is gone. The reason for that feeling is that your desire has been met. Your thoughts are no longer on the attack to fix the problem of life not aligning with your wants. In contrast, the negative on the stick ignites every cell of your existence on fire with sadness and overwhelming disappointment. Then the loop of *I am barren, I am barren, I am barren, I am barren, I am barren, I am barren* will play on forever. Pain is winning, growing, and not letting you go. You are mindless. You cannot see. The ego is one hundred percent in charge.

If only someone could have told me how to stop the loop. In order to stop the loop, all I needed to do was recognize the repetition and ask myself if it was true. To understand it, I had to become aware of my thought process. I wrote them down so I could see them clearly. What was I telling myself? Did I really believe what those thoughts were saying? Is this truth or fear generated from the situation creating the pain? The pain was caused by not being able to have children. I was in a constant state of dreaming about the want of children. I would wash the dishes and look out the window to see a child run past the house. My gaze would drift off as I dreamed about what it would feel like to have a baby inside me, driving home from the hospital, late nights staring at the newborn in amazement, learning to live in our new life as parents...all the things. But because it wasn't happening, the loops responded to all of this with thoughts of failure. The dream and the reality were not aligned.

The single most important moment of my journey was when this particular loop stopped me in my tracks. *You will never experience the whole point of female humans living on this earth: to procreate, to give birth, to mother.* I became aware of what this particular loop was saying by asking the question. *Wait a second, could this be true?* I sat with this for quite some time. I carried great pain for this thought because, at times, this thought was true for me. It is our birthright to bring forth children into this world. So yes, there is much truth in this. Is this what I will choose to define me? Or was a greater force trying to tell me the truth that I refused to believe?

Becoming aware of this loop by stopping and asking questions of my own mind was the beginning of my true healing from this nightmare. There is much power in questioning your thoughts. My perception was beginning to shift. One day, after reaching the top of one of my favorite mountain hikes, I nestled into my meditation rock, carved with a perfect indentation for sitting. I looked out over the green valley below and sat in deep thought; a gentle breeze swirled around me as a few crows cawed above. There was beauty in the stillness of the silence.

I will not let the pain of infertility define me and ruin my life.

I sat up and held my shoulders proud in response to this thought.

I am aware!

The loops stopped. Bearing children is not all there is in this life. There is so much more to dream, achieve, create, and manifest in this big, beautiful world. Now, this feels good and is something I can get behind. The positive of this awareness brought back the connection of my true self and switched my thoughts from mindless to mindful. The awareness of self-preservation became greater than that of failure. I smiled all the way back down the trail as the crows followed me, cheering me on my way. I still had a long way to go, but this was the first step to freedom.

UNWEAVING THE THREADS:
Belief Systems, Mindsets, and Reactive Loops

"If you change the way you look at things, the things
you look at change."

Wayne Dyer

One early morning before sunrise, I immersed myself in the internet, seeking insights into the mind's inner workings and thought processes. I stumbled across a spectrum of mindsets that fit in either the positive or negative.[10] Negative mindsets consist of themes of without, distrust, ineptness, failure, someone else is the problem, ungratefulness, entitlement, lack of passion, finding no meaning in life, and pessimism. In comparison, the positive mindset holds beliefs that everything is possible, passion for life, connection as one, accountability, gratitude, abundance, the power of giving and living in the present, and the power of now.[11] *I must be positive, right? I only have two from the negative list, so I must be all right then. I am not any of these negative words, except for the without and failure parts.* My desire was to align with the positive, yet internally I was tethered to the negative by sadness.

The fact is, we are conditioned from the very beginning by our surroundings and upbringing. This conditioning shapes our belief systems. This is important in understanding how our opinions are formed, how choices are made, how we interact not only with others but with ourselves, how we decide to feel about an experience, and finally, what we tell ourselves about it. How you were raised and what influences were given to you at the time of the pain trigger will determine how you decipher the information experienced from a difficult situation.

Ultimately, your mindset and overall belief system will navigate your way out of pain. But it doesn't make it any easier because grief is so challenging and heavy. Grief is associated with the negative because anger, cynicism, and sadness lurk close beneath. To me, grief and pain are one and the same. How we respond to pain becomes the key to getting out of it. I realized that I didn't want infertility to break my spirit forever, and in the depths of all those heart-wrenching moments crying on the floor, I felt broken. In search of how to answer that, I had to find something positive out of this. I chose resilience. Recognizing your mind involves acknowledging these various mindsets and consciously choosing where you want to stand on these opposing spectrums.

At the age of five, a cherished memory of my Grandaddy remains etched in my mind. I can still picture myself sitting beside him on the front porch during a Texas-sized thunderstorm. On that hot and humid day, the moldy smell of the old brown outdoor carpet permeated every corner of the porch. The thunder was rumbling in the distance but getting closer. My eyes were wide with a little fear as each crack of the lightning grew closer and closer. Grandaddy must have sensed this.

"You know, there are cats and dogs up there fighting in the clouds right now," he said to me.

I looked up at him with my big green eyes as my legs dangled and kicked lightly against the bench.

"Sometimes God is bowling up there, too," he added.

I grabbed his strong hands as we watched the storm come in.

After a bit of silence, he said, "Never let your desires overrule your better judgment."

I looked up at him with utter confusion on my face. These words were so big; what did they mean?

"You know those mini Snickers bars you like so much?" he asked.

"Yes!" my little self responded with a smile. It's candy time, my prize.

"You know how you feel bad in your belly when you eat too many?"

I thought about it and shook my head in agreement.

"That's what that means. When you want to eat another one, and you know you shouldn't," he stated.

How did he know I wanted another candy bar? I will never forget those talks on the front porch. These moments I hold close to my heart. These are my earliest memories of shared belief systems imprinted on my mind.

Since my mindset beliefs were set in the concept that I could do anything, when the reality of infertility took over my thought process, I moved into the mindset of failure and shame. I mean, WOW. This mindset was completely one-eighty from my core belief system. Without my knowing, my mind was being challenged by this failure of conception. *Why am I not getting what I want? I can do anything!* My mantra was not working, and I was surprised when it turned negative. *But you can't do this. You are a failure. This is a moment of shameful existence.* Thanks, loops. For me, one of the biggest reasons infertility pain is so difficult to get out from underneath is because the emotion of the pain was challenging my entire belief system. My I-can-do-anything mindset was compromised, and I had no idea during the heat of the struggle that this was happening. This is why I was confused.

Which mindset do you best resonate with between negative and positive? By becoming aware of your mindset, you can begin to process and understand how you are going to perceive the pain of the situation. If your mindset rests on the negative end of the spectrum, then the healing will be filtered through a running script of negative thoughts. If you constantly tell yourself you are not good enough, *this will never happen; just give up already,* then this perspective will be a more difficult terrain to navigate. The more you tell yourself these things, the more you will believe it, the more you will feel it, and the harder it will be to get out from underneath it. You will become overwhelmed by this feeling. The positive outlook will not be any easier when processing pain, but the energy associated with positive thought patterns will be more uplifting for the sadness. If you are having a tough day and you tell yourself, *it's going to be alright, you've got this, one day at a time, this feeling will pass, hold on,* then you are at least giving yourself a chance to feel good. You ultimately are the one to heal through this. No one else can do it for you.

With that said, there is no quick fix to any of this. The challenge is learning how to live through these experiences. Being aware of your belief system is key to developing and understanding the ultimate mindset to survive through pain.

Within a year after my periods stopped and six years into the journey, I was working on a production job at the Sundance Mountain Resort in Utah, filming a Suzuki car commercial, when I had an a-ha moment. It was an early morning start; we were getting ready to shoot as the sun was rising. We were up on a mountain pass, and the sun's rays were gold, pink, and glorious, a Kodak moment that took my breath away. In the silence of soaking in the sunrise, I heard these words: "You've got to deal to heal." I was lost in the beauty of the first light of the day, and it felt peaceful and right. I knew I wanted more of that feeling, to feel okay.

You've got to deal to heal. Huh. Easy enough, I can do that.

To me, dealing was doing the work to heal through the pain. However I could get there, I was going to do it. I knew it was going to take work and study of myself. Life was giving me a lesson, and I had agreed to learn with it to release the pain, verses ignore it and stomp the pain down in my belly, to fester and boil and feed the Void until I died. I did not sign up for that life.

I found a keychain at the gift shop at the resort made of a leather strap and a silver pendant, engraved on one side with a spiral circle and the other side said the word HEAL. This would be my keychain until the learning was done.

But how do I get there? All I knew was I wanted out of the pain. I wanted to feel good. I searched for anything and everything that would make me feel good. It's as easy as reading a book, watching videos that focused on positive affirmations, and tuning into Instagram feeds that reflected the state of mind I wanted, to the simple things like dancing in the moonlight or turning my favorite song up loud in my car with the windows rolled down. I found comfort in reading *The Four Agreements* by Don Miguel Ruiz, *The Universe Has Your Back* by Gabrielle Bernstein, *The Power of Now* by Eckhart Tolle, *The Secret* by Rhonda Byrne, *A Return to Love* by Marianne Williamson, *The Untethered Soul* by Michael Singer, *The Book of Awakening* by Mark Nepo, and *Many Lives, Many Masters* by Brian Weiss, to name a few. Through reading these words and filtering my social media with positive affirmations, I at least was able to surround myself with the positive. Even if I was not aligned with this positive feeling a hundred percent, and some days I was downright emotionally in the gutter in the negative, I knew the positive words were there waiting for me, like my dogs waiting for me to come home after a long day away. The mindset can change when you surround yourself with supportive information that benefits your well-being. I was learning that if I combined this information with meditation and intuitive thinking, I could shift my mindset.

INTUITIVE THINKING

"The intuitive mind is a sacred gift, and the rational mind is a faithful servant. We have created a society that honors the servant and has forgotten the gift."

Albert Einstein

Carl, the healer, was the first to tell me I was using my mind to understand how I felt about infertility. My mind was the first tool used to interpret the problem. Then my heart would react in some emotion to match what the mind had created, and my solar plexus or "gut intuition" would respond. The lines of communication were completely off balance. If you let your mind decide what the deal is first, then use your heart followed by gut instinct, you are opening yourself up to a whole range of randomness, given the complexities of your mind. Those thoughts are determined by your belief system and mindset. If those are off, then your entire sensory system is going to falter based on that first step alone.

When Carl first told me this, I was confused, as I had never thought about my energy receivers this way. Of course, my mind is processing how I feel; that's what it is supposed to do, right? I remember sitting in my aunt's living room as he told me this and placing his hand between my gut, heart, and mind. He said while touching my forehead, "You see, you have been feeling from here instead of here," as he touched my belly. "You cannot get the truest sense through your mind's eye, not like you can from your gut instinct. This section of your body is designed to hold nerve sensors that present negative and positive responses based on how you feel or sense the situation." I could understand this, as I had experienced these gut responses before in my life. What he was telling me began to make sense. I was letting my mind dictate the emotions with the negative loops. *You are a failure because you can't conceive.* Then, my heart would respond with sadness and feelings of anguish. My gut would follow up with no message at all as the proper channels were not followed. It is intuition that truly guides us. When we allow the mind to dictate how we should feel, then we are not allowing our intuitive nature a chance to support. Honestly, the mind then heart then gut sequence completely wipes out the role of our instincts. Your mind is already made up about how it wants the emotional reactions to flow.

What if we perceive through our intuition first? Then, our perception would not be based solely on what our mind's eye sees, which is influenced by our belief systems and shaped by conditioning. Our intuition, our gut, does not have a mind of its own. There are no thoughts running through our bellies to persuade what we are sensing. It is a knowing from within, a feeling, if you will, without the need for conscious reasoning. Simply put, a part of this knowing is based on past experiences and the other is based on trust. Intuitive thinking is sensing using energy vibrations to refine the response to the situation. Like walking down the street and passing by a person who gives you the heebie-jeebies—the hair stands up on the back of your neck, and you feel uneasy. This is your instinct, a warning sign has been given on an invisible layer, and you just know to move away from that person. Then you continue walking down the street without another thought other than *that guy was weird.*

Once this impression has been received from the environment, which is typically defined as good or bad through the gut, the heart delivers the message, and feeling is applied. Intuition will tell the rational mind where to look next. This truest sense of feeling allows the mind the space to process and understand the pain logically, outside of fear and panic. The rest of the body then follows, based on what the mind distributes as the reaction.

The mind left on its own to decipher how to respond is a weapon for disaster. My mind was often wild and unpredictable because it kept generating worst-case scenarios about my childless life that left me overwhelmed, sad, and panic-stricken. Once I allowed myself to perceive through my intuition first, feel the knowing with my heart, and let my mind understand it or define it, then I was able to surrender to the pain and begin to learn from it.

The irony of intuitive thinking is the part that is influenced by past experiences. With pain and suffering, usually this experience is a first. It is not like you have a recall about infertility, as if it has happened to you before. *Oh yes, I have done this before. I know how this will go.* The fact is, we don't know—and when you don't know, the best thing to do is let go and trust.

Chapter 8

Unlocking My Toolbox

"The quieter you become, the more you are able to hear."

RUMI

TOOLS FOR THE MIND:
Meditation and Therapy

Much like the tools needed to get pregnant—books, needles, bloodwork, sonograms, sperm cups, thermometers, and ovulation charts—tools are needed by the mind. Meditation found me about a year after my periods stopped. I was at a restaurant, nestled up to the bar, when I noticed the guy next to me had this blissful look. I thought, whoa, this guy has peace. I want some. Maybe he was smiling because of all the beer he was drinking, but nonetheless, he was there to give me a message. I couldn't resist.

"Can I ask what you are smiling about right now?"

"I just learned how to use Transcendental Meditation. I am doing it right now as we speak."

I later learned that you can actually do that, but you are clearly not as focused when conversing with someone simultaneously. This was intriguing. Why had I not thought of meditation until now?

I found a local class and signed up right away. After a weekend of in-person transcendental meditation training by a certified teacher, on the last day we joined together in the basement of an old insurance firm where the classes took place. There was a window between the dark office and a beautiful, light-filled atrium with plants. While the room felt dingy and trapped in the seventies, the life of the atrium illuminated, providing grounding energy to the group inside the room. We all sat in a circle and meditated together. This was my first time meditating with others, so I was uneasy, as sharing silent intimacy with strangers was quite foreign to me. However, as I relaxed into the moment, I began to feel the buzz we were sharing with one another in our energy connections. Even though the older man sitting next to me had a light purr of a snore, it did not phase me, and I was able to stay in the practice. I realized at this moment how the power of connection is so much stronger than one individual. The buzzing I felt was such an elevator of energy that it left me no choice but to leave the room feeling centered and balanced. I instantly wanted more. Meditation has the innate ability to calm endless mind chatter. It is a tool to promote well-being and exercise of the mind. Our minds need this just as much as our bodies. Had I realized this while going through treatments, I believe there would have been a better chance to succeed.

Meditation has been the greatest gift to find. I strongly suggest finding the technique that is right for you. There are many apps out there to help you learn the art of meditation. Whether you are in the thick of infertility or climbing out of another pain trap, meditation will start you in the right direction to get outside of your mind. I was so full of anxiety while going through the IVF treatments. Had I found meditation, I would have had a fighting chance to be calm through the process. Same with all the two-week waiting periods after procedures. I was never calm; I was panicked the entire time in the fear of *what if this doesn't work either, then what?* By quieting the mind, even for five minutes, the thoughts running wild come to a rest. The brief or long break is enough to quiet the mind and allow space for your soul to shine through. This opens the door to your peace. When the mind is relaxed, then the inner guidance of your soul has room to connect to your mind and body. Once this happens, then you find balance, and the dance between mind, body, and soul can begin. This dance brings healing, emotional understanding, and the creation of our best selves, no matter the negative outside factors that try to get in and win. The soul always shines the brightest, as this is who we truly are. We are not our minds.

VALIDATION SESSIONS

"The wound is the place where the Light enters you."

Rumi

Am I really okay now? I searched my mind often with this question. I would ask this and then wait to see what feeling I felt about it. After ten long years, I finally reached a point where I just felt nothing as a response, but not nothing as in the Void; this nothing was different, it felt peaceful. But I wanted to make sure. When I looked toward therapy at this stage of the journey, I knew I was seeking reassurance. I wanted validation that I had processed the pain correctly, if there is such a thing. I did not want the emotional scarring from this experience to define me, to be one that I could never get away from, like a bitter old woman scowling at energetic children playing in the park.

Whether I liked it or not, I had changed, but not defined by the pain. If I had attached to the feelings of infertility and not let go, then the negative influence of that feeling would have guided my mindset in how I functioned and experienced life. The result would be defined as a negative vision filled with bitterness, anger, jealousy, disappointment, and, ultimately, the loop of never being good enough. This was one hundred percent what I did not want. My experience changed the direction of my life in that it showed me the path of spiritual growth earned from self-discovery. Had I been blessed with the two-point-five kids and the family life that goes with that, I would have had no time to reflect, to go inside and try to manage the emotion of pain and digest, dissect, process, and eventually learn how to survive through one of life's greatest challenges.

Because of these defining thoughts and the residual heartache present, I checked in with a therapist about six years after I stopped trying to conceive. In my mid-forties now, I felt like I was in a good place in my heart since I wasn't crying every day and filling my mind full of infertile thoughts. I found a therapist who specializes in infertility. I actually thought about therapy for months before I connected. My hesitation was based on my preconceived idea that the therapist would have no clue what I was feeling, that it would end up pissing me off, making me feel even more isolated. How could they know without experiencing it first-hand? They can study all day long about infertility stress, but if they had not lived it, I had a hard time believing they would be able to offer me anything.

Finally, the day arrived and I made my first appointment, on my birthday. This is the one time of year that I am the most emotional about the loss. It is not on the anniversary of my miscarriages. Honestly, I can't even remember those dates other than spring, fall, and winter. It is my birthday that triggers me every year. I think it's because I am turning another year older and my birthday is in the spring, which is a time of renewal. That, and the fact that birthdays are a time of reflection. What I try not to do is reflect on what I am not, what I am less of. I do not allow that loop anymore.

Three things that made therapy successful for me were the timing, being open to it, and finding the right person. To me, checking in with yourself through therapy is a healthy way to support your mental health. Also, I wanted validation that I wasn't fucked up.

I actually laughed out loud as I drove that snowy April day to my first appointment. I talked to myself in the car. *Here it is, my birthday, and you've chosen to speak to a therapist about infertility? Are we ever going to be over this?* Her office was in a medical complex from the late seventies—angular roof lines, brown everywhere for siding and trim. The hallways were long and white with brown carpet and hollow doors, but her actual space was filled with a plush white couch lined with lime green and white pillows surrounded by light canary yellow walls. There was an oil diffuser dispersing lavender essential oil that was pleasant and not too overwhelming.

In that first session, we established our boundaries: who I was, who she was, and what I was there for. My sessions lasted for six months. I talked through all the areas of concern: the loss of self, womanhood, isolation, grief, bedroom issues, societal pressures, and how I have processed all of this. As I ran through the gamut of emotions tied with each of these features, she nodded and prodded with some questioning, but the prod was geared toward validating what I had experienced. It felt good to self-reflect. To look at the pain objectively while not controlled by it and to see that I had come a long way in my healing journey. The support of therapy is a gift, and when you are ready, take it.

When I am in the place of observation, I can see my thoughts come and go. Here, I am able to witness them pass by. It is like watching them appear on a chalkboard and then flowing across the board, disappearing when they reach the edge. I call this the zoom-out approach, where

I step back from the emotion and the sensations to detach and get a different perspective. This approach helps me become a witness. When I am observing, I have a chance to see whether or not the thoughts bear any truth.

One example of catching a negative loop in action came while walking through my house—putting away clothes, feeding the dogs, and making the bed—with my mind running a hundred miles an hour, looping about all the bad things of my life. Then, the emotion of overwhelming grief would show up. *Man, this feels like shit.* That right there was my red flag, and I stopped what I was doing and listened. I stood in my living room, took a long, deep breath, and then acknowledged my feelings. I even said it out loud. "Okay, yes, this feels like shit."

I reviewed the thoughts that were running through my mind and then questioned them (it helps to write them down and look at them). *Your life is done.*

Wow? Do I really believe that? No. There is great power in simply telling yourself *NO*. When I did this, my mind would stop the diatribe. This is how I eventually quieted the negative mind.

Okay, well, today may suck, but tomorrow will be better. Hang on.

I found this to be true because those words felt better. By the next day, the moment had passed, and I did feel a little lighter. The more I did this, the fewer grief moments I endured until one day, they no longer showed up. This awareness opened the door to a new understanding of myself. The ultimate truth I learned is I am not defined by my mind or my mental processes. I am the one observing them. This is when I got my mind right.

With my loops under control, I was able to receive the emotion of hope in a new light. Hope is always in your heart while wishing for your child. There are no other heavenly connections like faith and hope to bring forth your desires. When failure overrules hope in relation to infertility, you ultimately begin to lose hope. And when you lose hope, you lose everything. My new thought of this-pain-will-not-define-me and what the miracle of that awareness meant to me was that my life, in itself, is the miracle of hope. I had lost hope. Truly, when there is no hope, you will find yourself on an isolated path. There is no more connection. It is just you and the loops until the awareness of them changes the path. While my pain did not disappear overnight and took years of work to complete, this shift in thought was the beginning of getting out of the pain. When I focused my energy on mindfulness, then I knew I would win this battle of self-destruction.

The pain of infertility will not ruin my life. I will have a wonderful life without children.

And you know what? My mind will be okay with this. I will be okay because the tool for surrender is to stop trying to control the outcome. Releasing this energy for control made room for strength and compassion to enter back into my heart, and for surrendering the burdens of infertility.

Chapter 9

The Healing Meter

"Healing doesn't mean the damage never existed. It means the damage no longer controls our lives."

AKSHAY DUBEY

Her long, blonde hair was twisted in a loose braid to one side. She wore a white tank top that showed off every curve of her round pregnant belly. I didn't know her name, but she caught my eye as I waited to cross the street. There was a slight breeze as I watched her sitting contently on a bench outside the ice cream truck, enjoying bites off her ice cream cone. She was smiling between bites as she held her belly with her left hand. She seemed so at peace at that moment, happy.

I was deep in my journey, not trying to conceive anymore, mid-forties, when I found myself standing on that street corner, as a single tear rolled down my cheek beneath my sunglasses. I quickly wiped it away. This told me the pain was still there because I was still feeling sad when I saw something I wanted. But it was lighter because I only produced one tear. I crossed the street and went on my way to finish my errands. This trigger was different because the pregnant lady did not bring me to my knees, pushing me to drop everything I was doing and run away to hide in my car and cry until the pain passed. It only got me a little bit this time. That's when it hit me.

Am I ever going to be done with this? When will I be healed?

I needed some sort of way to measure where I was on the spectrum of healing. I was so tired of experiencing these surprise triggers. I thought if I could have some sort of way to check in with myself, to measure the pain and how I was feeling and reacting, then I might be able to be done with this. I wanted there to be an ending. I imagined the emotional scale went something like this: "real fucked up," "still fucked up," "sorta fucked up," to "I'm good." Naturally, I created my own measuring tool if you will, which I called the healing meter. This was like my internal compass, analyzing my emotions and reactions. The heart of the healing meter was becoming aware of how consumed I was with the problem. Did it take over all of my thoughts and feelings, and how often? Since I had discovered the loops and the power of my mind, the healing meter centered around this awareness.

When I first thought up the healing meter, at this point in my journey, I felt like I was somewhere between "sorta fucked up" and "I'm good" because pregnant ladies still got to me. Otherwise, for pretty much the entirety of my journey, I was in the "real fucked up" to "still fucked up" stages. To me, the meltdowns and the crying dictate where you are on my fucked up scale. The more I worked through these emotions, the healing meter soon developed.

The healing meter has three parts: Observe, Accept, and Transform. Observation is key to understanding your feelings, which measures how often you cry, how intense your breakdowns are, and how much time you spend thinking about infertility. Once you move past this stage, you move into acceptance, enabling you to let go of the pain and allowing room for you to transform and grow as a person. This is the path of healing and growing through it. But in the end, it really boils down to when you stop freaking out.

OBSERVE

The first measurement was to monitor the number of crying episodes, specifically tracking how many times a day, per week, and per month I was spending energy on crying. In the beginning, I cried several times a day, every day, for a very long time—years. Then it became a couple of times a week, and then eventually, I would save it up for monthly emotional meltdowns. The meltdowns felt like setbacks because they were so full of anger and rage that drained me emotionally. They made me feel like I would never heal. I guess I had more freaking out to do.

Then one year, they stopped. All the triggers that fueled the meltdowns (pregnant ladies, babies, asking if we had kids, baby showers, self-limiting thoughts) no longer worked. This was one hundred percent due to my mindful practices and work on becoming aware of the loops. I meditated twice a day, every day. I was able to connect with my thoughts and learned to observe them here without connecting emotion to them. The thoughts no longer controlled my feelings. I got to decide whether or not I believed the loops. Any damaging thoughts like *you are a failure because you can't have kids* were not accepted. I now questioned these thoughts. *Really? Do you REALLY believe that statement?* Through meditation, I was able to calm my emotions.

Once I was able to see my thoughts, I was able to let go. This awareness was the game changer. When the meltdowns stopped, I knew I was one step closer to the "I'm good" stage. The pain triggers no longer served me, for when I was observing first, I gave myself the space not to believe them anymore. I had cried, yelled, pleaded, and sat with it long enough. You are done when you decide to be done. It's when the analysis is complete, and there is no more data to digest. The mind has finally looked at every single angle possible to understand and make meaning of it all so that closure can occur. It's almost as if the mind decides it is no longer interested or has grown rather bored with the content, and then, just like that, the pain stops.

Today, pregnant ladies remain my gentle reminders. Even at forty-nine years old. While getting ready for my workout class, as I stretched in the studio, I watched as the instructor took a photo of another cute blonde wearing tight black leggings that showed off her perfectly round belly, as the pregnant lady posed on her toes with one hand in the air and the other resting on the bar.

I put my leg up on the bar to stretch, rotating my right shoulder and laying my arm out over my leg as I turned and watched this scene.

There she is, a pregnant lady.

I switched legs and continued stretching. I smiled at her and the excitement she carried for her pregnancy. I did not feel sad, jealous, or envious. I felt joy for her, and I could feel her joy. And that was it. I went back to stretching.

I'm still okay.

When I was in the "still fucked up" stage and getting to know my thoughts, I focused on how much time and energy I was spending each day thinking about infertility. I finally got to a point where I rarely thought about it. I was amazed that this was even possible. I would find myself on a hike where I used to think about getting pregnant and my emotions the entire hike, and realize where I was now. *Wow, I didn't even think once about infertility.* Eventually, I reached a point where my mind didn't draft a single thought about infertility for entire days, weeks, and even months. That's when I knew I was close to acceptance.

ACCEPT

In order to fully accept being childless, I had to let go of the dream. I couldn't get past this because of my belief system: try hard enough, and it will happen. I desperately wanted to be done with this story. To be able to mean it when I told myself, *I'm good.*

How do I let go of a dream?

Dreaming is how we move through life and create. We dream about our future, where we will live, how we will spend our time, what work we will do in life, what adventures we will find, and who will be with us. If we want to make a change in our lives, we dream of something new. Dreaming is our creative process, our paintbrush for creating a new idea into a reality.

Then there is the universal dream, the dream of family, marriage, and children. It is our job, our God-given right, to bear children, be mothers, be fathers, and continue the dream like so many others before us. The universal dream carries an enormous magnitude of expectation and is one of the biggest reasons infertility causes such heartache when you are not part of this dream. It's big.

In order to let go of this infertility nightmare, I had no other choice but to accept defeat. I had to look at my wishes, my desires, and my dreams of raising a family and set them free. I couldn't hold onto them any longer. We will not be parents in this lifetime, period. *Accept that.* No amount of heartache, pleading, and God talks will change the ending, ever. I lost for the first time in my life, in a big way.

"Trust in the journey," God reminded me.

So, what did I do? Ten years in, I held another ritual in my meditation room for the final release. I'll admit, there was to be more crying, but I knew in my heart this would be one of the last moments of emotional release in order to get to the end. I created a sacred place, surrounding my altar with the loving energy of rose quartz crystals, and burned sage to clear negative energy from the space. I sat cross-legged in silence on my vanilla-colored carpet. *Thank you for this journey. I am grateful for the wisdom this challenge has opened to me.* As I opened my pain mind, I looked back and allowed all those emotions that had driven me to hell and back to show themselves again. As I ran through all of them, I observed their level of control, if any, to measure how my body felt as I sat through the memory of the pain. Where was I feeling pain in my body, if any? That's what I was looking for—for the measure.

At that moment, I was able to clearly see the spectrum of emotions and see myself sitting within all of them, from disbelief, anger, sadness, guilt, blame, anxiety, and depression, to acceptance. I could see myself in each phase of "really fucked up," "still fucked up," "sorta fucked up," and "I'm good." I moved through these feelings without a reaction from a safe place of observation. Then, I sat in silence before fully releasing the dream of having children. I acknowledged all facets of the experience from a place of peace. I spread out my right hand over my heart, pulled my fingers together, grabbed the energy out of my heart, and threw it back to the universe to dissolve and disperse into healing light and joy. This was my physical way to let go of the dream. When I was done, I closed the door to my meditation room, and let go of the dream forever. What I learned is that once the dream leaves your heart, you can let it go.

We are never truly done healing, as the insights continue to grow with time. We become a greater version of our old selves from the wisdom gained in the experience. It is about how you choose to respond. For me, it was about learning from my mind. Once I figured out how to observe my thoughts, my world changed. My thoughts no longer controlled me, and this was freedom. This was the only way out of pain. The power has always been in the choice.

Even though my personal belief system was exploited when I was not able to use my decision-making to will a child into my life, I did not let infertility tear it completely down. Once I got through the confusion and shock of this, I was able to accept that I do not have the power to bring forth a life, even if it's what I deeply want. I cannot make any decision or choice to change this. *Accept.* What I did have control over was the power to choose in my response to one of life's greatest adversities.

Connection: The Retreat

About a year into my infertility struggles, I picked up the book The Infertility Cure by Dr. Randine Lewis, but I wasn't ready for it. It seemed like so much to do to try and get pregnant. It was an alternative approach and ironically felt more intense than the Western medicine way of drugs, blood work, shots, and IVF. This approach was overwhelming to me because deep down, I was pissed that I couldn't get pregnant the old-fashioned way by just having sex and calling it good. The concept of The Infertility Cure was to nurture the body to create an open and inviting womb for the soul baby by tuning into diet, herbs, and acupressure through an ancient Chinese wellness program. After the IVF treatment failure, I decided to pick it up again, now five years into the journey. Nothing else was working, so why not?

I read the stories of women just like me who were becoming pregnant by following Dr. Lewis's guidance of caring for body, spirit, and mind. My focus now had shifted to mastering everything Dr. Lewis had to say about infertility. I was her newest pupil, and I was going to succeed through her methods so that I could become a testimonial on her website.

As I read her work, I was focused on what kind of deficiency I had. What kind of herbs should I be taking? Vitamins? Fish oil? As the book suggested, I wanted to make sure my acupuncturist knew exactly what my body needed, even though what I was asking him—or better yet, telling him—to do was somewhat against his own unique wisdom. There was a specific diet to follow, the Spleen Qi diet. I wasn't entirely sure what it was about, but I tried to follow it. No wheat, no dairy, no cold drinks, no sugar, and no processed food.

I kept going back to the website, scouring through the testimonials, feeding what little hope I had left. What caught my attention the most were the stories of how amazing the retreats were and that one must attend to truly understand The Infertility Cure. The next one was to be held in Austin, Texas, at a healing center. My mother urged me to go and even gave the retreat to me as a gift. I was reluctant about going because I didn't want to sit around crying with people I did not know. I had done all the treatments, and nothing worked, but I still had hope for a miracle. Focusing on my body, mind, and spirit was the only thing I had left. This was a chance to connect with other women about the struggle and hopefully learn something new.

I arrived at the retreat in style after an hour's ride from the airport in a smoke-infested white sedan. I was more comfortable with a car service than a stinky cab, and Ubers did not exist yet. This car service was accurate because it was my life mirroring my current condition: trying to mask my spirit body with a fancy car service that turned out to be the exact opposite. Maybe I had not healed completely yet.

The retreat was held at a healing center built high above Lake Travis, nestled in the treetops. The accommodations were heavenly. I had my own private patio looking out into the surrounding woods. There were several buildings sprinkled throughout the complex, including housing, the dining hall with a limestone balcony overlooking the lake, the full spa, several halls for group gatherings, and a serene library with floor-to-ceiling windows surrounded by the woods. There was a meandering dirt path consisting of labyrinth energy, with sections of the trail hidden by Texas mesquite trees.

I arrived a day early as I wanted to acclimate myself and settle into the environment. The place had a peaceful feel to it that I resonated with instantly. I felt calm here. The first night was about meeting for my initial consultation with one of the acupuncturists. The consultation was in one of the guest rooms with rich red curtains and a cozy blanket on the bed to match. The windows and walls were trimmed with heavy wood, and the room felt organic and in sync with the woods that surrounded the center. The acupuncturist I met with was Liz. I entered the room, and she asked me to sit on the edge of the bed as she ran through the standard questions: how long have you been trying, how many times have you been pregnant, have you ever tried acupuncture, how many treatments have you had, what's your current diet structure. I responded very quickly with annoyance because, to me, this was my résumé of failure.

Liz took notes as I spoke and was very serious in her evaluation. I was almost uncomfortable. Am I signing up to be all I can be right now? This was more like an interview with a drill sergeant to join the Army.

"I have to ask," she says. "Do you smoke?"

What an odd thing to ask. Do I smell like smoke? Why on earth would she ask me this? Did she mean marijuana? I was almost insulted.

"NO! Like now? I mean, I used to smoke a pack a day."

Then she stared at me as if I was lying. Could that be the reason why I'm infertile? Did I poison my ovaries and eggs with nicotine? Then, there was a more uncomfortable silence while she continued to stare.

Oh my, we are not getting off on the right foot. This is going to be a very long retreat for me. How do I get out of here?

"It's just that I have a keen sense of smell, and I can definitely smell smoke on you." Again with the stare.

I stared back. I darted my eyes.

Are they going to let me into the retreat, or what? I don't smoke!

Then it hit me—the car service. "Oh! I know, I know, I rode in a stinky car service today filled with smoke, and the button was broken to roll the window down."

There was silence and staring before she spoke again.

"Interesting. Well, smoking would obviously not be helpful in your situation. Let's move on to your treatment for the evening," she answered, not believing me.

I had been seeing an acupuncturist specializing in more traditional Japanese methods, so I was alarmed to experience the Chinese version. The difference is in the Japanese way, needles are inserted and then removed in an instant, but in the Chinese way, the needles stay in for a half hour or so while you lay and meditate or relax into the treatment. I was unaware of this, so I sort of laid there in the hotel room with needles everywhere, wondering how long I was going to be there. I eventually relaxed into it.

"Your energy is grounded," she told me. This made me feel good as a confirmation that I was getting better. At this point, I was trying to feel good again. I had worked hard over the last year to get out from underneath the suffocation of grief. I came into the retreat believing that I had more pain than everyone else. I was certain of this. Not sure why I felt the need to measure this, but I did.

The acupuncture treatment was wonderful. I was relaxed, and my energy was zingy but calm. I showered right away when I returned to my room. I tucked my stinky smoke clothes in my bag. I sat on my bed in my minimalist guest room with hardwood floors, all-white bedding with navy blue throw pillows, and journaled as I drank a cup of hot tea. I was more than excited about what the first day of the retreat would bring.

The next morning, I got up and got lost running on the trail systems. A misty fog was in the air, and the run seemed magical. As I made my way down the meandering trail through the woods with tree roots crossing over the path and the morning birds singing, I imagined how I would introduce myself. I recounted my story, the miscarriages, the treatments, the sorrow, and then, as I turned my thoughts toward the reason I was here, I could feel the sadness begin to awaken and rise to the surface. I was here because I was determined not to let infertility ruin me emotionally. Tears ran down my face. Great, I haven't even started the retreat yet, and look who is crying already, alone on the trail talking to herself. I really must be a lot crazier than I thought.

But this cry felt different. It was a sweet victory cry of who I have become—a woman of strength, courage, and hope. Here I am, standing in her truth, no matter whether the outcome is welcomed or not. This is who I am. This is whom I will introduce to everyone at the retreat.

The next three days were amazing. I met wonderful women whom I could connect with and talk to about the emotions of infertility. It was healing not to feel alone. And I quickly realized my pain was not any greater. We were all in the same grief. For the first time in a long time, I felt I could exhale and feel normal amongst these new friends. The retreat was filled with tools to support the mind through meditation, labyrinth walks, a burning ritual to release what no longer served us, education about diet and supportive herbs, wonderful healing meals, and how to perform acupressure on ourselves and each other to support the body, mixed with a ton of sharing of our stories and feelings, and finally the ending ceremony for our spirit.

Shaman music played softly as we entered the healing center with our shoes left at the door. The room was lined with floor-to-ceiling windows met with dark wood floors, surrounded by the greenery of the bushes and trees outside that engulfed the center. There were thirty of us, and we lay in a circle with our heads toward the center. Dr. Lewis asked us to hold hands to complete the circle. I had no idea what to expect as I had never been in any kind of healing ceremony before. I had to truly go with the flow as I lay with my heart open and mind free of words. Several healers in the room performed reiki, acupuncture, acupressure, and aromatherapy. These healings were done individually and then as a whole in the group. My eyes were closed, so at times, any one of these healers would rotate through and add a needle, perform reiki, or dab my head with rose oil. I could feel the feminine energy of the group running back and forth through my hands. This was the first time I had felt energy in this way. It was like someone plugged us in, vibrating and rolling between and through us. It was real, and it was powerful. There was crying by all at different times, and when another would cry, you could feel it in your heart.

Then, my stomach started to rumble. Uh oh. I might have to poop. I became distracted and worried that I was going to have to get up and go poop and ruin it for everyone else. No, you cannot get up and poop right now. You don't have to poop. But the feeling was not going away. I knew it was nervous energy because my mind was taking over. Damn it, Shannon. You are going to wreck this whole experience. STOP IT.

And then the most amazing thing happened. I tuned into this nervous energy and accepted it. My body relaxed as I moved into this energy at the base of my spine. With my eyes still closed, I squeezed the hands of the woman next to me and allowed this energy to move. It became a spiral and began to swirl and gain power. Then slowly, it rose up from the base of my spine to my belly button, to my chest, to my throat, to my eyes, and out the crown of my head. It cleansed my soul as it rose through my body. I no longer had the urge to go to the bathroom. Instead, I was vibrating, more like buzzing at a high rate, and my body, mind, and spirit were one.

When the energy left my crown, it felt like an explosion of release as I moved into oneness with the universe. All I could see was the black of the sky and stars. It was quiet in there and peaceful. It just simply was. While I was still connected in the healing circle with the women, I was floating in this other space of the universe. Then, my son appeared in a field of wheat with blue skies all around. He looked to be about eight years old, and he had tan skin and long, sun-kissed brown hair just below his ears. He had beautiful green eyes, and he was happy. His name was Joshua. I got all of this information downloaded in an instant. He was running toward me through the wheat field and laughing and smiling. My heart was full as I watched him. Without speaking, he told me with his eyes: it's okay, Mommy, all will be okay. My heart swelled, and tears rolled down my face as I exhaled all the worry and sorrow from my heart. The ladies to either side of me squeezed my hands. I wanted to stay in this field with him forever.

The ceremony ended and signaled the close of the retreat. The ceremony lasted for about an hour, and when we came out of it, each of us had a serene glow as we smiled and looked at each other with our hearts. Something happened that day; something shifted for each of us. I later learned that energetically, I had a Kundalini awakening. That was the swirling energy I experienced climbing out of the base of my spine.

I carry that ceremony close to my heart to this day, and I can still see Joshua smiling at me in that field. The retreat changed my life and helped me connect again. To know that there is support out there. It helped me work through the pressure situations that were to come after. It was the toolkit I would pull from on my way back to me as I continued to grow spiritually. It gave me great peace knowing that Joshua was there; he will always be there. Ultimately, I found connection with myself through self-discovery and embracing vulnerability.

TRANSFORM

Then there was the Thanksgiving of 2018. I have to admit, here I am in the middle of writing this book, thinking that I've got it made in the healing department, and then WHAM, out of nowhere, and I mean literally nowhere, the pain sneaks up on me. I seriously had not cried in years about this. Now, I question whether I have much more to heal than I thought.

I could feel the pain start to well up in my chest as we sat around in the Vrbo rental with people fairly new to me. While I had mostly met these people through weddings and funerals, they were old family friends of my husband's family. They also all had children, all of them with two to three kids each. No one knew my story here.

At first, I felt fine. *I've got this.* I have been in these situations time and time again. But a few things were lining up nicely for me. First, a comment was made earlier about someone else's life while on the car ride to the Vrbo. "What life? She has no life. She has no kids and no grandchildren." That stopped me in my tracks. I instantly thought of myself and my life (even though this was not directed at me); how could I not stop and contemplate that statement?

Is that how I will be viewed when I am seventy?

The real issue is that, while the person who made the statement didn't think twice about what was being said, it was the start of a minor meltdown. My mind latched onto it. Sitting around the long, wooden farm-style kitchen table, laughter, wine, and funny stories were being shared. Then the conversation turned to what everyone's children were doing in school, sports, etc. I sat in silence. Drank a sip of wine.

I took a deep breath and could feel that sliver of pain rise slightly.

What is this? A bit surprised that I am really feeling anything at all. It had been so long, but I recognized the Void.

Uh oh. This might not be good, I told myself as my eyes got a little wider.

Smile more, I told myself as I put on a fake smile, clenching my teeth. Then I thought of the words from earlier, "No life. No kids. No grandchildren." *I don't have any of these and never will.*

Gulp. I poured myself another glass of wine.

More outward silence. *Is this conversation about kids ever going to end?*

I did my best; I went to the bathroom and looked at myself in the mirror.

What are you going to do about it? You are writing this book to help people, and you can't even help yourself at this very moment! The emotion had taken over and overwhelmed all normal brain activity. Sadness was now there, but no tears.

My husband had no idea what was going on with me at this point; in fact, no one did. But I knew how to get out of it. I began to question. Why am I feeling this way? What has happened that has overwhelmed me? For one, the no-life comment was made. Two, we are in a social scene and connecting with people I barely know. These conversations are completely normal for people. In this case, it was Thanksgiving, two families reconnecting that had grown up with each other. All the other families have children. As the children ate sugar and ran wild throughout the house, every few seconds a Mom would reach out and grab one for a quick few minutes of bragging rights—more silence from me while on the inside, I carried on my thoughts with myself.

Smile, take a sip of wine so no one knows.

You know what, no one here cares that you don't have children. They also have no idea the pain you have suffered, and that doesn't even matter.

I was in complete shock that this was happening to me again.

Am I really feeling this way right now? I mean, I have definitely been down this road a thousand times. How can I possibly be feeling this way at this point in my journey? Is the healing meter failing me?

Even though the emotions boiling up were the same, I was responding differently. I was aware. I was fighting hard inside not to let my thoughts walk me straight into the Void. I was aware of my thoughts and how they were making me feel. While I was not able to turn them off as soon as they developed, I could see them, and I was observing them. I wasn't angry with the person who made the no kids, no life comment.

Don't react to what you are thinking right now. Observe. There it is. The healing meter is working. Finally, the night ended, and we headed back to our hotel.

When we got back to the room, I jumped in the shower because I felt like warm water running over me would wash away the feeling of isolation. As the emotions of the day washed down the drain, the tears fell in a steady stream. I let all the thoughts from the evening replay as I took a deep exhale and let them go, one by one.

No life. No kids. I will never be a part of the dream.

Then I stood in silence until my husband ripped open the shower curtain to see me crying. I turned away and cried what was left of my mascara into the towel draped over the shower rack. I told him all the things I had been thinking about and how the no-life comment got me. I stayed in there until the loop stopped, and the pain subsided.

I can do this. There will always be holidays. There will always be society everything. There will always be families with children everywhere. I fell into the bed naked, curled up with my body pillow, and drifted off to sleep.

I was fine the next day; the rest of the holiday was great. I had made a clear choice of what I wanted for my experience. I could have continued down that no-life road and had the worst time possible, all from my own doing. I would have sat there and not engaged and secretly been angry about kids running around being happy little beings. Instead, I got to know everyone, talked to them about their lives and likes, and yes, even child-rearing.

In fact, when the kids would get wild and scream, I made light of it and said (in the most playful way), "Whose kids are these screaming? Would the parents of this one please get it under control?"

And the group actually laughed, and you know what? I felt accepted, kids or no kids. I chose to be engaging. I chose to participate in what life was showing me at that moment. I chose my reaction. My reaction did not choose me.

A few days after I returned home, the one who made the comment shared with me a sweet photo of myself and two littles as I showed them a funny animal app on my phone. I could see from the photo that I was okay. I was not sitting off by myself and unavailable. I realized that you don't really heal from emotional trauma. *When will I heal and be done with infertility pain?* I had been asking the wrong question. What I should have been asking is, *What will I learn from this?* A deep, emotional wound is a road to wisdom through great suffering. Therefore, what you become after is a transformation of self through the wound.

So, how do you know you have reached the "I'm good" stage? It's all about how you feel, determined by less crying, less desire to be alone, acceptance of self, less negative mind loops of without, more connection, and the desire to engage in life occasions. This is what feels good. This is your meter to tell you life is okay; you are okay. The reminders will always be there to show how far you've grown. See them for exactly that, and then let them go.

The year before my fiftieth birthday, this happened. There was something small sticking up from the freshly cut grass in the middle of the fairway. I noticed it as I walked up to my next golf shot.

I leaned over to get a closer look. "What is that?" I said to my friend, who happened to be infertile like me.

And there it was, a white pacifier with little sailboats on it, right there in the middle of the fairway.

I smiled and let out a chuckle, "You know what's funny?" I said as I picked it up and held it in my hand, "I used to find these all the time, and I would save them. I took it as a sign that the babies were coming." A memory flashed before me of when I found one in the alleyway by my downtown office. I remember vividly how it made me feel back in the "still fucked up" stage.

Let it go.

I tossed it in the golf cart as I walked back to my ball.

"But that ship has sailed. And I'm good with it."

And I meant it one hundred percent.

Chapter 10

(Waving the) White Flag

"If you allow it, suffering can be the means
by which God brings you His greatest blessings."

CHARLES R. SWINDOLL

As I stood on the stage, I crossed my left hand over my heart and pinched my nose closed with my other hand. I turned and looked over my right shoulder to see a few people sitting down below in the audience. The lights were bright, so I could not make out any faces. The balding pastor draped in a white robe was saying something out of the Bible. I don't know exactly what. He had his hand on my head as he spoke. The people below could not see the light blue kiddy pool from Kmart behind me. All I knew was that I was "supposed" to be doing this to get saved. I was fourteen, while all the other kids there were under the age of ten and were also getting baptized that day. I was only "half in" to this idea that dipping me back into the kiddy pool with a dead black cockroach floating in it would actually save me from going to hell when I died. This is what they said to do. They being the people who went to church. Curious, I had been going to church with friends, and after a summer church camp in 1987, I decided that I would do it too—the herd mentality at its finest. I wasn't raised in a traditional go-to-church every Sunday family. In fact, we never even talked about religion in the house. Didn't pray before dinner or bed either. My family left this part up to me and allowed me space to figure out religion for myself. So I gave in and trusted the bald man to hold me as he dipped me into the roach-infested waters. I didn't feel much different after the water washed my sins away. But the small audience clapped below, and the people around me smiled and seemed relieved they had saved another poor soul from the depths of hell. After that experience, I can't even remember the next time I went into that church. I never carved out time for Sundays, really. I didn't see the point, and without pressure from my family, I just left that baptism right there that day. Felt more like something I checked off my to-do list. Baptism. Check.

Ironically, years later I found myself in a spot left with nothing else to do but pray. It was three o'clock in the morning, when my thoughts were so loud they practically woke me, running at Mach speed. Great. My heart was racing, and my thoughts were consumed with replaying everything that pissed me off from yesterday. I sighed and then counted, but this did nothing. I tried a new relaxation trick, counting three deep breaths again while thinking of the word "relax" with each exhale. That did not work. Still, the thoughts were rampant and irritating. I changed my position in bed, from side to side, to my back, to my stomach. I took a sip of water. Nothing was working, and I had finally reached my last resort.

In my head I said these words.

God, are you there? Can you please calm my heart rate and help me fall back asleep?

I waited. I did not become instantly relaxed, and I heard nothing back. In fact, my heart rate was up so fast that I felt heavy in my chest and thought I might have an early heart attack. As I lay there, my mind turned dark. *Maybe this is why I am not to be a mother.* I'm scheduled to die young, and that is the reason. I had thought this several times, but at this moment, I felt maybe that's why I should reach out to God even more.

I waited some more. It dawned on me while I waited for God to clearly answer back in some sort of George Burns-type voice: *Do I even know how to pray? Does God really want to help me go back to sleep? Is that the right time to pray?* I mean, I have prayed in my lifetime and several times during this baby ride, but I have never prayed every day. I have given a silent thank you for gratitude on days when I felt great about my life. I have prayed for those who have died, even for people I didn't know and had read online about their untimely deaths in some tragic accident. To me, I felt like these were good things to talk about with God.

Give me a sign to move on. Help me accept that I will not be a mother and will still have a beautiful life. I surrender! Help me to learn joy and gratitude in other ways. What I did not ask was for the blessing of a child. I had squashed the desire to have a child because it wasn't working, and I was angry about it. I felt I had to turn the desire off in my heart to protect it; otherwise, it felt like it might stop beating. So I didn't even think to ask for a baby.

"Shannon, pray every day. Why not pray for a healthy pregnancy and see what changes may happen?"

I could hear the voice clearly in my head. The voice was deep and calming, like Morgan Freeman. It was like being wrapped in a warm, cozy blanket on a cold day.

God, is that you?

"Yes. Accept. Pray. Let go."

This is your advice?

"Yes, then write about it. Get up right now and write."

What about that work email from yesterday?

"Does it really matter?"

No.

"Then let it go. The pain is there to teach you to let go."

I proceeded to tell God about the abortion I had at age eighteen, and I told the unborn child that I was sorry for ruining our sacred contract. Then there were the souls of all of the miscarriages.

I'm sorry, souls, that my body was not good enough.

By the time I was in year seven of trying, I had already buried the desire of a child so deeply that to dredge this feeling up from the depths of my soul scared me. I don't want to be obsessed with this anymore. I want to be accepting of my situation. Even though I was forty and the clock was very close to burning out, I still had the desire for a child. I still dreamed of a miracle surprise pregnancy. What I wanted to know was which way to go. Do I stop wanting the baby now? Can I simply turn that off? Show me a sign, please.

God, I need a break from the heartache part; that would really be a welcomed relief. I am so tired of these murky feelings. Please help me to feel the desire again without the despair of looming failure attached. Is that even possible? I have no idea how to do that.

"Allow without fear," God said.

Fear of what?

"Fear that it will never come true. What will it mean if it never comes true?"

I shifted my head to the side of my pillow toward John and sighed.

It will mean that I will not be a mother.

I had a strong belief, and I could envision the miracle pregnancy. I always had a vision of being in my early forties and reading the pregnancy test, seeing the two lines, running to John to show him we finally did it, watching my belly grow, and ending with holding our newborn in our arms. This belief held true for me until the clock stopped ticking.

Crap. I'm getting old

That, and I hadn't had a period in a year after age forty. Since my periods changed and seemed to be gone, I was getting the message loud and clear that my time was up. The window was closed, and it was time to accept reality. That is the reason I decided to let my desire go. It didn't make any sense otherwise. It only deepened my sadness, and there was no sense in wallowing in things you cannot control. It was time to let go. But this little piece of hope that lived deep inside of me was hanging on, that something good was coming my way.

God, I pray for your guidance. I don't want to keep going down a path that leads nowhere. Time is running out for me and in my wishful thinking of getting pregnant, even without a period, and in my heart I know this is not going to happen. I am at the end of the road. I am ready to accept my path, but with less heartache, please? Maybe I can talk my body into having a period again? I don't even know if I am praying right. I will keep trying. For now, I will focus on allowing without fear, however that happens.

"Now you are on the right path to surrender," God said to me.

While this was a gentle wave of relief, it was mixed with sadness as reality became, well, real.

I was still not ready to get out of bed. A gentle rain began to fall on the roof in the early morning light. I was finally able to relax for a moment before my mind scanned again and reminded me of a recent conversation I had with my best friend.

She said, "Your biggest problem is that everything you have ever done in your life, up until this point, has come so easy." She was right. Everything had come easy to me. I could make my career, my marriage, where I live, my play, whatever I wanted, happen easily. If I didn't like something, I changed it.

Trying to have a baby was the first time something was not easy for me. After our conversation, I sat with this idea for a long time and then finally reached clarity on the core of this concept. The law of free will does not work with infertility. This was my conundrum. This was my struggle. We are conditioned to use our will to make decisions in life. To obtain goals, you dream, you figure out the direction needed to build something, whether a job, college, building a career, volunteer work, climbing Mount Everest, or whatever drives you; this will to succeed in that experience is what gets you there. The tool we use to create is manifesting, attracting the reality we wish to create. Some things fall in your lap, and some you have to work a little harder for, but this is our birthright, the gift of free will.[12]

How can I have the ability to manifest my life so easily in other areas, but now it is not working to conceive and have a baby? As I questioned this concept for years, I one day connected with the idea of free will. If I have free will, then so does the unborn child. What if the spirit baby changes their mind at the last second? These ideas began to change my perspective. It brought clarity to me as to why this struggle was so frustrating to me. You cannot will a baby into this world because the soul coming in has its own free will and choice of when to come here. No amount of willing, wishing, dreaming, manifesting, or stomping your feet will get that baby here. It's all on their time. The laws are simply not the same between manifesting and conceiving. Manifesting does not include the creation of a human being, period. We manifest to create a reality that we desire and, in doing so, attract that reality and then use our free will to guide us on choices that reality presents to us. If another human being's path aligns with this reality, then that is how they are brought into your manifestation. There is no such thing as control in this process. This is based on our free will and the destiny tied to the experience on a spiritual level.

Was the destiny of my life meant to be childless, and was I manifesting correctly not to conceive? Then I remembered my vision of Joshua from the healing session I experienced at the infertility retreat I had attended. What about my dream baby Joshua? Was that real? Was that my destiny, or just a dream? He was definitely our child, and this vision kept me connected in hope that he was coming. I desperately wanted to understand what was behind the curtain to be learned from this pain. I didn't have the answers; all I had was nothing. What I didn't have was control. It was time to get out of bed and get on with it.

A few days later, I was on a walk with my dogs after dark on a full moon night. I love full moons in Montana. They light up the skies as bright as day. As I watched the dogs run and dance off and on the trail by our house, splashing in the creek and surprising a sleeping duck, I realized that the tools I had used to navigate my life were not going to apply to having a baby. I could not control the outcome. The only thing left to do was surrender.

"I have no control," I said softly out loud to no one. I looked up into the light of the moon, the Milky Way sparkling around me, and with tears in the corner of my eyes, I whispered up to God.

Did you forget about me? I have nowhere else to turn.

"Good, that's what I wanted," he said.

At some point, I was told along the way that infertility does not exist in Heaven. This comforted me as it made sense. Our loved ones are there. Joshua is running through the fields there. Our furry friends are there. Life is there. If infertility does not exist in Heaven, why not view it that way on Earth?

Once I fully understood that my way of manifesting did not apply to conception, I began to step aside and connect with my unborn child's soul. I began to honor the soul for its journey. I slowly changed how I looked at "having" the baby. My focus was on getting something, like a new car. I had been going about it the wrong way the whole time. I made it all about me and had lost the connection with the spirit baby. Secretly, I still had hoped this was going to work out.

I had no particular "style" when it came to praying. It was more a conversation in the car, in the shower, lying in bed, hiking the dogs, and sitting on top of mountain tops. But these were the words that came with the most power.

I need help.

Show me the way out.

I give up.

I spent a lot of time alone, contemplating all things infertility, and prayer usually happened most of these times. The more I prayed, the more I fell deeper into surrender. Something about the act of asking was soothing. The energy of surrender actually brought me some relief. I found that the act of talking to God opened the doors of my heart, and in return, my healing began. Through this act of praying, I was inviting healing energy into my life. The worried thoughts started to retreat. The familiar panic, shame, and sadness now had a competitor as love was fighting its way back in. It is love that picks you up off the bathroom floor. At first, surrendering may feel like giving up, and in some ways, you are, but not as you might initially perceive. What I was learning about surrender is that I was giving up the internal fight, which brought an end to the negative loop cycle of abuse. This was my White Flag moment, permission to let go of the hurt.

As I began to accept that I would not become a mother, I felt the next step was to make amends with my unborn children to bring closure. In my case, I felt there was one, maybe two. Soul contracts are between souls before they incarnate into a physical body, like an agreement of how we are going to work together. Whatever our soul contracts were, I needed to release them from the contract. There is no handbook to follow. The guilt I carried for breaking one of the contracts led me to perform a ritual to release the spirit baby I had aborted at eighteen.

My husband was out of town, and I had the house to myself. It was winter, and the snow was falling gently in the dark of night. I had the fireplace on, my favorite candle lit, and I burned palo santo to clear the energy of the room. I arranged a comfortable spot in front of the fire, filled with pillows and my preferred soft blanket. I poured myself a glass of red wine and set the mood by turning on the sounds of a gentle rain from the playlist. This sound is calming to me and symbolizes the clearing of energy, washing it away. I lowered the lights. My intention was to create a warm, cozy, safe place to make a heart connection with my spirit baby in my living room.

I was told in a reading by a woman who specializes in connecting with baby spirits that my spirit baby hangs out with me on my left shoulder and has been with me since I was a little girl. That was comforting to me and also very sad to me that I denied this one's birthright to a body and life. But I hung onto this reading that I needed to connect and release the spirit. There are no instructions for this part either, so I went with what felt right to me at the moment.

I took three deep breaths and focused on the flicker of the fire. I centered my mind and allowed the thoughts to float by without attachment as I slowed my breathing and tuned into the energy of the stillness. It is here that we can connect. I took another deep breath in and waited. My mind had flashes of the abortion mixed with visions of what my life would have been like had I kept the child. Images of Joshua would flash. Then, I relived all of the losses, the abortion, the miscarriages, and the dilation and curettage (D&C) procedures. The tears began to flow. I allowed this moment and gave the spotlight for all the emotions and feelings just to be, to release. I didn't need to hold onto them anymore.

I am sorry, little one, that I did not hold up my end of the bargain. I love you very much and always will. If you have a chance to have a life with another family, then so it is; our contract is released.

I laid my head down on the pillows and cried a very long and deep cry. When I was done, I burned the palo santo again and spread the smoke all around me, especially on my left shoulder. I sat in my scene for hours in a quiet state of being. When I was ready, I blew out the candles and went to bed.

I still had questions for God. Why am I not fit to be a mother? Am I not compassionate enough? I'm short-tempered and impatient. That would make a terrible mom. I get annoyed easily. I'm irritable. Really, when I think about these thoughts, I laugh out loud because all of my mother friends sometimes feel like this. That's life, and some days that is motherhood. Yet still, the question lingered. My heart was so frozen in stone from the protection of pain that I couldn't feel compassion anymore. I had lost it from my heart. People would tell me their life pain, divorce, death, or loss of some kind, and I would feel nothing. It felt like that to me because I had so much pain in my mind and body that there was no room for empathy for others' pain. I really had no sympathy for what they were feeling.

Maybe that is why I am not a mother. I am not compassionate enough.

In my search to understand why, I realized this question was the driver of my pain and kept me connected to the story. This gave power to the loops that often pushed me toward life comparison with others. This was dangerous to my self-esteem.

Why them, not me? Why do the crack addicts have babies and not me? Why?

"You signed up for this. It's your life lesson," God reminded me.

Wait, God, what does that mean?

Is he telling me this whole experience was meant to be? As I moved deeper into the solace of surrender, these new thoughts showed up for me to push me into acceptance. As I felt this new belief system coming to me, I could see the lives lived before this lifetime in meditation. This sight was more of a knowing. I was a mother. I was a mother many times before, and I didn't sign up for that in this life. When I really sat with the question of why, these were the answers I got.

My granddaddy always told me, "If you don't know what to do, then do nothing at all. When you wait, the answer will come to you." So, I returned to this mindset. I did not know the answer as to what to do next. The only message I was receiving, loud and clear, was that the answer to bearing children was a hard no. It was obvious when my periods stopped.

The end of my cycle was the beginning of my true healing journey. When I turned to God for help, my cycles stopped. That is exactly what I needed to stop the hemorrhaging of defeat. I am grateful that was the ending. What louder sign could I have received? Once my cycles stopped, I started shifting the desire to conceive to healing from the experience. It would be the healing of the aftermath that would take more time.

My mother answered the question if I was compassionate enough. I shared with her my thoughts on my internal introspections. She said to me, "Yes, you are; look at what you do for your dogs so that they can have a good life. You are always thinking about how to take care of them. That is compassion for another being other than yourself." She was right. I probably spent way more time thinking about their well-being than most people, some might say a bit OCD at times, but that was my way. If I weren't compassionate, I would not care about their well-being.

She got through to me on this, and I was able to stop letting my emotions be controlled by the thought of *you are not compassionate enough.* That is not the answer to the why. The answer is and continues to be that having children was not meant for this lifetime, period. The experience of not having children was absolutely what this lifetime was meant for me to understand. As I sat through this new wave of thought, the more I began to understand the implications of what life was trying to teach me, the more I was able to let go. Little by little, I was beginning to see the light at the end of the tunnel. God was there.

God was listening. I needed only to listen back. I needed to ask for help in the first place.

"I am always here."

You see, we all have a plan, a learning lesson from our lives. While the plan is not always made clear upfront, this is to aid in learning the lesson. The hard part is putting trust in the whole process. Trust in the journey to move through it, for if there is no journey, there is no growth. All of this is needed to experience life. That's how we experience it, and the whole reason for great pain is to trigger growth on a spiritual level. This is what God was trying to tell me.

With this new awareness, it was time to grow past the pain. I had been working on understanding pain's emotions and how they affected my overall well-being. I needed to understand this process in order to move past it fully. I believed this understanding would set me free from the loops. This pain taught me to use my heart, connection to God, and life to get to the other side of healing. Closing myself up and hiding in the pain from others was not the answer. These pain lessons were presented to aid me and remind me of my connection to spirit. They were painful because I was using my mind to heal versus my heart. That is why they are called heart lessons. This is healing.[13, 14, 15]

"Allow and accept."

Through acceptance, I began to open my heart to God. A new hope showed up for me, not attached to motherhood. This was a hope of happiness rewarded at the end of the lesson. I had longed for my old happy self. I would often think back to a time I was happiest, and it was on my wedding day. I was overwhelmed with gratitude; at that moment, life was pure, easy, and perfect. Our whole lives were ahead of us. That was me before the pain, but I recognized I could never get her back again. I was to become something greater.

"Welcome to acceptance." Love, God.

Chapter 11

Life after the Clock Stops Ticking

"The only journey is the one within."

RAINER MARIA RILKE

Life continues, and in my pursuit to move forward on my own terms, guided by my newfound beliefs and self-awareness gained from my infertility journey, my focus shifted to a few key elements that helped shape my new mindset. These elements included being mindful of my intrusive thoughts, nurturing myself to find personal fulfillment, seeking to connect with other travelers on the infertility journey, cherishing the bonds with my niece and nephews as part of my family circle, and prioritizing attention to my marriage. This fresh outlook was and continues to serve as my personal support system, guiding me to grow through the trials of the pain.

Catching My Thoughts

Long after we were done trying, one hot summer afternoon, the skies grew dark as another thunderstorm rumbled to the west, preparing for the arrival of a heavy rainstorm. With the front door open, I sat on the front porch as the metal wind chimes swayed gently back and forth, playing a soothing tone. The wind shifted and changed energy from a gentle breeze into intermittent blasts of wind as the storm rolled closer. In these moments, I am fully present. It's hard not to let the mind wander when engulfed in Mother Nature's wonder. The smell of fresh rain in the air, a slight drop in temperature, birds chirping, and the subtle hints of flower essence from my hanging flower pots all brought a feeling of peace.

As I nestled into the cushions of my favorite outdoor chair, my mind began to self-reflect. *It's been more than ten years, and look at you now.* I took a breath in. *You are okay now. You have accepted fate.* And I wasn't crying about it anymore, either. I was just there, sitting in acceptance. I guess you can say I was feeling pretty good about life. I reflected with a smile as I observed my current state of mind. *You did it. You survived this.* As I sat in silence with this thought, almost proud of myself, my mind decided it was a good idea to give me a little test to REALLY make sure I was good. Instead of savoring this peaceful moment, my mind went on a walkabout. Why do we have to take a perfectly good moment and turn it into something else?

Out of the blue, I looked to the future. What about high school graduations and sending the kids off to college? These normal life events are coming next. I could see the graduation announcements pouring into our mailbox for our families and close friends' children. There would be celebrations for the graduates, and while we would enjoy being a part of the festivities and cheering on the young ones toward adulthood, I also saw my husband and me standing off to the side in silence, squeezing each other's hands. This would only be a reminder that we have no child to celebrate milestones for. As the thunder rolled across the sky, the rain began to fall as it was building up to full power. I found myself holding my breath tight. I hadn't thought about this part. *Well fuck, am I ever going to get away from this tragedy of life?*

Of course, my mind did not stop there. I wanted to know more about what the future may look like. *What about engagements, marriages, and grandchildren? Oh my God, grandchildren. I can see it now, all of our friends and family as proud grandparents showing off the new addition to the family all over Facebook. What the hell am I going to do?* I sat in silence as I listened to the rain, now a heavy downpour filled with cracks of thunder as it ripped through the sky. The smell of wet grass and dirt floated in the air.

The storm was directly on top of us now; the sound of the rain beating down on the roof was deafening. I continued my way through the landscape of my life, and there it was—the ending. I saw myself alone, my husband long dead, and me having to move into a stale white-walled nursing home. I imagined clearing my home, life possessions, and what I would do with them. I have my great-grandmother's silver. I have my grandaddy's Dutch cooking pot, my grandmother's button of the blue dress she wore to my wedding, my mother's baby photo and lock of hair, and lamby pie, my mother's baby stuffed animal. There is no one to take these. That is just it; there is no one. What about all of the things that were mine and my husband's, the things that we cherished? There is no one. I can only hope that my niece and nephews will care enough to help, but they may not. So, there I sat contemplating the end, and I began to cry. For that vision of life, alone with literally no help, is very, very sad.

The storm had now rolled past the house and over toward the next town. I could hear the thunder off in the distance, the dark clouds following, leaving behind a light rain as the rays of the sun streamed down through the clouds. Still holding my own court, I pulled out of the future and realized how each phase in life would be impacted without children. Since we had made it through the beginning stages of children with our friends and family, I thought we were good. We could handle not having children. It wasn't until I imagined my entire life and all the milestones that make up all of our lives that I realized the magnitude of not having children was on pieces of our lives. It's not like you didn't get a job that you really wanted. Not having children affects your entire life, all facets, till the very end.

I was in shock. *How will I survive? Not just this moment, but my ENTIRE LIFE? I am never going to be able to get away from the barren title. We will forever be isolated from everything in life. I will have no idea what that feels like as a parent or grandparent.*

As I processed this, I began to plan for the future. I was more concerned for The End than anything else. I did not want to be a burden to my nephews and niece. That meant I had to plan and have all of my belongings donated to a church or other local community that needed them. The things that meant the most to me, like my crystal collection. If not, let it go and donate to an organization that would want it. I would mark the most precious items to us so that they knew. Like the petrified bonsai tree, a gift from me to my husband for our fifth anniversary. Suppose I have to live in a nursing home—then that bonsai goes with my husband—or if I'm left alone, it stays with me. I will plan the funeral, so all they have to do is call—no decisions to be made. I'll leave a list of any friends who may still be alive and need to be contacted. I will make sure my funeral music playlist is played, the most important part of it all.

The planning calmed me down. The birds were now chirping in the sunshine, the storm had long passed, and I could feel the wood beams under my feet again. *It will be okay. I will be okay. This is all a part of life.* Being a burden on anyone is a common reaction, whether you have children or not. The alone feeling I had dreamed up for the end—with no one to care about me—was a vision of great sadness if I chose to look at it that way. I let my mental storm pass, stood up, and made my way back into the house.

Envisioning life milestones without children is a part of the healing process. When it comes up, recognize that focusing on the alone part of that vision will only create negative thoughts, bringing the focus back to the empty dream. Allow the thoughts to transpire as they will, but don't engage as if they are real. Don't get trapped in the sad emotion of being alone like I did on the porch that day. No matter what stage of your life, children or not, being alone is a real fear. We are not meant to be alone out there, and that really is the trigger in this particular vision, not the fact that there are no children to bury you. While yes, that is obvious, you can't count on anything in this life as a given. What if you have children and they don't speak to you? They don't care, don't visit the hospital room, and sell all your belongings without attachment to granddaddy's cooking pots?

The fact is, what happened to me on the porch that day started with thoughts of without and then merged into the emotion of sadness as my thoughts continued down the winding path of life moments where children should be. It is obvious that not having children changes your entire life perspective. But now, I choose to observe the emotions that show up after contemplating the "without" life, rather than let those thoughts determine how I should feel.

Honoring My Center

On day three with my healer Carl back at my aunt's house in Texas, we stood in the living room in front of the window next to the adobe fireplace my uncle built. I was watching the horses in the pasture when Carl said strongly to me, "Shannon, I want you to open your heart fully and think of joy. Think of love washing over you and filling your heart. That is all."

He put his hand on my head and took in a very deep breath. I instantly felt a rush of energy filled with pink and white light pour from him into me. It traveled through the top of my head and washed through my body to the tips of my fingers, down into my toes. The healing light then rose back up through my body, carrying all of the negative thoughts that filled my soul. Suddenly, this negativity was right in front of me, with thoughts rapidly running through my mind, word by word, reminding me of all the horrible things I had told myself about infertility. Every word I had ever cast upon my soul was lifted. The sensation was that of release. Carl's healing energy was able to insert the light into my being and reverse all of the control the thoughts of my mind held hostage over my spirit, and my body. He replaced the negativity in my body with light. This healing light took up the space that the negative was using. There was no place for it now.

"Remember, Shannon, the flow of life is like water. Think of the sound a river makes when it flows. All you hear is the water running. That is the flow of life, and it is just that simple. The head complicates things and creates scenarios and thoughts that are not true, and sometimes we get tripped up in that, and then the body follows. Life is simple. It was designed that way. We are the only ones that complicate it. It should always be simple, every step of the way. When you start to slip, think of the water and focus on that. Our energy should always run like a steady stream of water."

What he was teaching was a tool to stay grounded and a way to get back to me. I still carry the meaning of this healing today. Especially as I hike through the mountains with my dogs and walk alongside a creek. I often stop and tune into the sound of the trickling water and watch it roll and fold as the water meanders downstream, carrying a small leaf, dancing through the ripples in the glistening sunlight. Under the gentle sound of the running water, I hear these words of my healer, and this brings security and stability to my experience. Once we feel secure in our situation, we can begin to start something new. To be able to look at the pain and tell it, *Hey, you know what? I did it. I am still here. I didn't die on the bathroom floor!* Finding myself again allows me the freedom to start something new.

For the Love of Goat Herding?

If you could do anything in the world, what would it be? Our minds love learning something new and especially when it brings us joy. This is how we connect with the feel-goods in our life. I knew this was a much-needed step to finding my joy again.

I wanted to learn how to work stock (as in sheep, goats, and cattle) with my herding dogs. It was my first day of training with my eleven-month-old border collie, Bowie. The drive to the barn was only two miles from my home. With my country music blaring, I turned down the dirt road to the barn on a crisp October day.

Standing outside a small, round pen filled with goats was Barb, in her early sixties, a native Montana rancher, smoking a cigarette with her hair pulled back in a ponytail and a baseball hat on. She took one last drag before she pinched off the end and threw it on the ground to smash it out with her boot.

Sizing me up, she tilted her head and reached for my hand. "Hi! I'm Barb. Tell me what you know about working dogs."

I shook her hand and smiled, "Well, nothing. I've always had border collies and always wanted to do this."

I saw in the distance a large, round pen with a guy working cattle by himself. I tend to have zero patience, so I naturally wanted to be where that guy was, working solo on cattle. "When can I do that?" I asked.

Barb turned and looked at the large pen. "You mean work by yourself?" She said with a chuckle. "Let's just see how we do for today." She later told me that the first meeting made her smile, and she knew right then I would be a good student.

We set up lessons for once a week to start, then moved to twice a week on Tuesdays and Thursdays. We worked with goats at first because they are way more forgiving than sheep. They waddle as they walk, shaking their heads back and forth, and they don't bolt like sheep when the dog is too close. They are slower in their movements, not as edgy, and when learning this sport, you want slow because there are a lot of moving parts between you, the stock, and the dog. I often equate the sensation of working dogs and stock to rubbing your belly while backing up a trailer with your eyes closed.

The day it all clicked happened one day in the barn about six months into training. It was winter and it was snowing hard, so we worked inside the dusty barn to stay warm. The day was so cold you could see the particles from our breath in the air. The orange tabby cat sat up on the hay bales overseeing our progress.

I watched as Barb carried our favorite training tool, a stick with a flag on the end of it. We were learning how to fetch, to have the dog bring the stock to you. Barb walked in figure eights around the barn, she in front with the flag, the goats in between her and the dog. When she turned right, she would hold the flag in the air, which applied pressure on the dog to stay back, a warning. Then, she would pull it down and keep walking. The dog should naturally curve around to the left to hold the stock directly behind the handler, then fall back in line to be centered on the stock as he brings up the rear, if you will. If they get too pushy, you feel this as the stock runs you over or past you.

You can use the flag to block the dog's movement. If you don't want the dog to go in the direction he is headed, you swing the flag out to the left or right to block them. They see the flag, and that signals to them no, go the other way.

"You see what I'm doing here? I am blocking them from circling all the way around. We don't want that. Keep them behind the stock. Their job is to keep the stock together and bring them to you, not past you," Barb said as she moved through the motions. Then she handed me the flag. "Now you do it."

I got nervous whenever it was my turn because I wanted to get it right. I still was confused about my directions and the overall feel of it. Barb had a way with dogs; they knew by her presence not to mess with her. She commands respect instantly, and they respond to whatever she asks. When I step in, for some reason, Bowie seems to give me the finger and blow me off. He gets pushy, and the stock runs past me and over the top of me. Today, I literally fell face down in the dirt on myself, the flag buried in the dirt from the goat hooves.

I was pissed, angry, and embarrassed. "I can't do this," I yelled out at Barb.

"Yes, you can!" she yelled back. She also had a way with humans. She could be intense at times while training because she could see what you were doing wrong, and you would hear it clearly from her.

I dusted the dirt off my pants, got set, and started walking again. I mimicked Barb in figure eights. I turned right and raised my flag, then left and raised my flag. Bowie stayed behind and then pushed. In the past, I would raise my voice and very loudly say, "NO!" This only made Bowie more intense and run faster and disturbed my goats. The goats' eyes got big; they were looking around, wondering what was going on with the crazy lady yelling. But today, I turned calmly and walked through the stock behind Bowie, pointing the flag at his eyes.

My eyes glared at him, and he knew something was amiss. This tactic Barb taught me is what you do when the dog is pushing. I backed him off, glared at him, and said, "What are you doing? Knock that off." I was on to him, the timing was right, and he knew it. He backed off the stock and was respectful of not only me but the stock. I let go of my anger and kept going. Bowie and I were in tune with one another for the first time. He took all of my commands. I was able to down him anywhere in the barn, meaning the second I said down, he laid down and stayed. I was able to walk him up slowly to the stock and then lay him down again. I could switch directions, and he responded to my flag and did not push.

This was our first victory. We were in the flow. The animals taught me this feeling of flow. The only way to be in the flow is to be present in the moment. The key is not letting your emotions take over. This is mandatory to truly be in tune with herding because the animals are feeding off of your energy, both the dog and the goats.

I was fascinated by this connection and surprised at how the lessons of herding tied into my healing. To be in flow is to be grounded and aware of your emotions and your thoughts. In this awareness, you can step out of the way and into the flow of life with ease and without resistance. When herding, the animals project back your state of being, whether you like it or not. You learn to read their behavior and respond to you as a check-in to adjust yourself.

I had found my new thing, and my heart was full of passion; my mind was intrigued. Learning something new helped me to keep walking away from the pain. My focus shifted to what makes me feel good and happy. I'm gonna find that and do more of it.

Finding My Tribe

A big part of my self-esteem was lost from the social dynamics of not fitting in with all of society. There was never a way to escape it. You couldn't even hide in your house and watch TV because a diaper commercial or an insurance advertisement showing life from marriage to old age and all kids in between would come on. This part was like a big thumb squishing my heart into the ground.

While it wasn't the intention of our parent friends to exclude us as they lived through the war zone of child-rearing, we simply had nothing in common. Suddenly we realized, let's hang out with people without kids. I mean, if we can't join them, then join someone else. Not sure why this concept was so foreign to us at the time, but once we figured this out, our world began to change from a life without a community to normalcy again.

We planned multiple trips to Hawaii, Arizona, and the Palm Desert to enjoy the sunshine, hiking, golf, and beaches. We bought a 1989 Westfalia van and created a lifelong friendship with new friends and their van, camping all over the West Coast. We found our laughter again. This was the change we needed from the social isolation we shared. Once we found our empty nesters, we suddenly felt accepted back; our self-esteem was lifted. This new circle didn't care whether we had kids, what Thomas the Tank Engine books we had, or whether our kids signed up for T-ball or not. They were more interested in creating a friendship, something my husband and I craved and were missing.

Forging Connections

Looking back, there were a number of times I was able to help others struggling. Years ago, I found myself sitting with a good friend over a beer. I could tell my friend was agitated when I sat down at the uneven table at the local bar. She had a distant look in her brown eyes, one that I knew well. She cupped her beer with both hands and clicked her wedding ring against the glass; she said, "I know you and John have been trying." *Here we go. Don't cry.* I gathered myself.

"Yes, we have."

"We have been trying for six months, and it is just not happening. I don't get it; we do all the things, the timing, the temperatures, and still nothing. How do you do it?" she asked.

Instead of feeling like running out the door, I felt a connection. It was the first time I saw my suffering as a way to help someone else. While I was in year five of trying at the time of this conversation, it didn't matter; I could see the panic in her eyes, and she needed to talk about it.

"You will be fine; give it time. You don't need to worry at this point in the process. Now, when you get to where I am, that's when you really need to worry," I told her.

"I know that's what I am looking at, how long you have been trying. How do you do it? How do you not worry?" She asked.

I didn't have all the answers. But I had the experience of what I had been through so far. "I do worry. But it's all because of the time. All I can say is know that your journey will be unique. You may have to go down a similar road as me with tests and IUIs and IVFs; you may not. It may just happen. You have to stay open and know you will be okay in the end."

I didn't even know how to communicate this message then because I was in the thick of it. But soon, I began to see that sharing my hardships actually gave her hope. She could see that her situation was not nearly as bad as mine. Oddly, these conversations with friends made me feel better. They always came to me. My philosophy is that if I live through the suffering, I might as well share it to help others. Helping others who have silently suffered through infertility or pieces of it was essential for my reconnection to self-love.

The Favorite Aunt

When we stepped off the plane onto the tarmac in Belize, it was still hot as the sun was setting. I snapped a photo of my thirteen-year-old nephew as he took off his Nebraska Huskers sweatshirt. He could not stop smiling.

"How does it feel to be in another country?" I asked him.

"I love it. First time in another country. I mean, wow," he replied.

John and I made a promise to all our niece and nephews that at the age of thirteen, we would take them on a big trip, to teach them how to travel out of the country. Christian was our first kid to take abroad, and he chose Belize.

The next day we went on our first adventure to see Cahal Pech, a local Mayan ruin in the town of San Ignacio. The three of us were walking through the town and jumped in a cab. As soon as the cab started driving, I realized our mistake.

"Christian, we just made a mistake there."

"What?" he said with concern.

"We did not ask the driver what the cost was before we got in. You never want to do that. We also did not ask the front desk where we were staying or what to expect for the cost. You always want to do that." The drive was a fifteen-minute drive outside of town, and he charged us fifty bucks.

We had a great first day exploring the Mayan ruins. Christian climbed over and above, in and out, of the ancient stone and walkways. Then, it was time to head back. The cabs were lined up.

"Christian, ask the cab driver how much. Cuanto?"

He asked, and we found it was only ten bucks! "You see, we got had on that cab ride out," I said. Christian shook his head as he took a swig of water. "I'm only telling you this, so when you have a girlfriend and travel with her someday, you can be the man and take care of her. You will know what to do." This embarrassed him, and he laughed uncomfortably.

Being the favorite aunt actually feels pretty darn good. If you have nieces and nephews, be there for them. You are an important part of the family dynamic and can make a difference to them. Embrace this relationship and make the effort to be a part of their lives. While not the same as teaching your own, you can influence and support them to be their very best selves—a great reward to your heart.

My husband volunteered in a local program by visiting his assigned kids once a week at school. He played card games with them over lunch, taught them to play cribbage, and listened and talked about whatever the kids were willing to share. At the end of the volunteer session, the kids would send him thank-you cards. These cards meant the world to John.

Volunteering to help children is a wonderful way to give back and to feel like you are making a difference because you are. Give back to non-profits in the community, whether that be financially or with your time for programs that may need assistance. Giving is rewarding and will not only help that program but will help you reconnect.

Don't Forget about Your Partner

Connect with your partner. Everyone experiences pain differently. Don't get stuck thinking they need to feel the same way about infertility. This will never happen, and it is simply not fair to place that expectation on them. Our vows warned us about these times, and we promised to be true to them in good times, bad times, sickness, and health. There is no one to blame for infertility. The positive? You have all the freedom in the world to be with your partner, to play, travel, and enjoy your best life.

Say It Outloud

There is an incredible amount of healing that takes place when you begin to share your journey. Other than the few friends who asked for my advice, I never offered to talk about my struggle. I once thought about posting something on social media on Mother's Day. *Why in the world would I do that? I don't need a sympathy card from my social network.* But my book became the focal point as I neared the finish line. I knew it was time to talk about the concept of this book to my friends. Once I took that step, it opened up conversations about our story, and what infertility feels and looks like from the inside.

Of course, I had to go with this and tell my story on a microphone at a wellness retreat I put on with friends. I have a thing about microphones. For some reason, if I have one, it's like I am transported to the stage. The lights turn on, blinding my eyes for a second while I regain my focus on the audience. Then I am on.

The twenty attendees were sitting in a circle on the oak floors, waiting for my presentation. There were crystals and sheepskins and yoga mats spread throughout. I was wearing a wispy white shirt and pants that flowed with my movement. I was there to teach them how to use crystals for meditation. I was beyond nervous.

I knew there was a microphone in the room and had joked earlier about using it. But with twenty people, you really don't need one. With a shaky voice, I started my speech. "Today, I am going to teach you how to meditate with crystals." *I'm not feeling this. No flow.* I stopped and called for the microphone. "Seriously, ladies, I need that microphone." So my co-workers laughed and grabbed my magic voice machine. They knew how nervous I was.

"Testing one, two, three. You got to always say that when you have to use a microphone, right?" I said as the crowd laughed with me. Then, like magic, the bright lights kicked on in my mind, and I was on. These words just flowed like water through me.

"I learned about crystals and meditation to help me get through the pain of infertility." There, I said it, and I had them all engaged! *This feels good.*

Then, these words came through out of nowhere and were not what I planned on sharing that day.

"When dealing with great pain, you've got to ask yourself, why do I feel this way? Where is this coming from? And do I believe it? Take a good look at this and challenge it. Because there is a good chance that you are telling yourself something on repeat, and you believe it without stopping to ask if it is true for you. This is what infertility taught me." Drop the mic. This said it all.

The power in speaking your truth, that moment of truly standing within your creation of life, in all the good and bad, is liberating to the spirit. Speaking your truth not only helps you grow but also helps others grow. I will admit I was surprised to hear the feedback from so many that day; they had no idea we had struggled. I just assumed everyone knew because we had no children. But the truth is, they didn't.

By communicating and letting others know of my experience, I have been able to connect not only with women with infertility issues but with people experiencing pain in general. By communicating, we connect and gain strength from speaking our truth. This honors the entire experience and our growth from the lessons.

Under the bright lights of my bathroom mirror, fresh out of the shower naked and with hair dripping wet, I practiced answering the question, "So what's your book about?" And I fumbled through all sorts of answers like, *It is about pain and not getting what I wanted. It's about the bullshit of life that infertility brings. It's about the emotional rollercoaster I've been on trying to conceive and the death of a dream. It's about being pissed off at the world. Boy, you have a lot of work to do.* As I practiced, I would imagine the look of horror on someone's face if I blurted out any of these words, all with a smile, while we sipped cocktails at a Christmas party. I finally rehearsed enough and came up with this: *It's an inspirational memoir about surviving the pain of infertility.* I said with certainty to myself with my hands on my hips.

There. That's it. This is my coming-out party to speaking my truth about infertility. I practiced these words, making sure my voice was strong and not cracking as I pronounced them. This is my truth. I stand proud in this, for this is what happened, and I own every piece of it.

Vision Quests

I have a box wrapped in red satin. This is my dream box. It was time to dream something new and let go of the old dream of coming home from the hospital with my new baby. I bought a bunch of magazines, and with my red satin box, I sat on my king-sized bed surrounded by white pillows. *Now what?* I had never been in this spot before, like sitting in front of a blank canvas, but this canvas was my life.

I opened the box with nothing in it. I stared into it. I got nothing at first. *How do I replace such a big dream?* I flipped through the pages of the magazines. There was the silver Toyota 4Runner I always wanted. I'll start there. I grabbed the scissors, clipped the picture out of the magazine, and threw it in the box. Then, I saw the washer and dryer I always wanted, clipped that too, and threw it in the box. Next, I saw someone running and healthy. An image of a woman standing on top of a mountain at sunset. I grabbed another photo of a couple happy and laughing. Another travel photo over the ocean someplace. Next, I moved to inspirational words like contentment. If I couldn't find the picture, then I wrote it down. I am a successful writer. I received a $20,000 gift. I am a stock dog handler.

The material things were just little goals and things I wanted, but most of the images were how I saw myself in the future. I wanted this for myself, and how I saw my life without children as easy, happy, traveling, and comfortable. The new vision is more about being open to perceiving a life without children. By opening up to this new perspective, I found the groundwork needed to allow a new dream to develop. Through the powerful tool of visualization, I was able to harness the creative energy to make this vision a reality.

When we feel it, we believe it and become it, except in motherhood. I have struggled with this concept of dreams and manifesting what you want in life. On one hand, I believe that you can have anything you want out of life that can be created. Ironically, the greatest creation is life. So why can't I manifest that, then? What I have come to understand is this. You could not will or manifest another soul into your life if it were not predetermined on a soul level for your lifetime. There is no choice you can make to change that agreement. Or you can look at it as maybe the answer is that there is no answer, only acceptance of what is.

Once I was done with my new vision of myself, I closed the red satin box, placed my hands on top, and said these words aloud. *Universe, these are my visions for myself. My intentions I am setting to bring forth this reality into my life.* This process helped me come to terms with letting go of the baby dream. There are more dreams out there to imagine than the family dream. And yes, you can feel joy and completeness again, and you will.

Embracing the Unraveled Me

Then, one day in meditation I heard these words: *Your life is complete as it is.*

Holding my clear quartz crystal, surrounded by my plants, I sat with these words as I repeated them to myself out loud, "Your life is complete as it is."

Huh. What does this mean?

It is not rare for me to hear messages when I meditate. Often, I will hear something like this, leading to other epiphanies. In reflecting on my own question, I've come to the realization that having children does not constitute or complete one's life. I am the one who holds the power to make my life complete.

It was time to open to a new belief system of *I have all that I need*, and to believe and live this way. Every day, I would wake up and tell myself, *I have all that I need. I have all that I need.* The more I told myself this, the more I was able to shift and believe it. The single greatest lesson learned was to become aware of my thought patterns, period.

I am more powerful than the words in my head.

In the end, my most healing meditation came with this vision. It was a warm summer day, and I saw myself lying in my yard, resting my head on a pillow in the grass, with my dogs nearby, enjoying the peaceful moment. The bright blue sky shimmered above, as white puffy clouds morphed into various shapes, drifting with the wind. The temperature was near perfect. I became entranced by the clouds, and then I heard it: the fluttering of the white silk fabric, the flag billowing back and forth in my mind. I took a deep breath in and let out a long exhale.

Everything fell into stillness. There, I recognized what I had been searching for—the calm from that day on the mountain.

I raised the White Flag of my mind, heart, and soul to the sky. I envisioned it stretched out above me, fluttering in the breeze, the sunlight filtering through its shadows. The calm of surrender washed over me as I raised the flag high, my final offering, my surrender to it all.

And with that, my journey of pain changed course.

I smiled to myself with recognition.

I'm good.

"Letting go gives us freedom, and freedom is the only condition for happiness."

Thich Nhat Hanh

Endnotes

1) Ramezanzadeh F, Aghssa MM, Abedinia N, Zayeri F, Khanafshar N, Shariat M, Jafarabadi M. A survey of relationship between anxiety, depression and duration of infertility. BMC Womens Health. 2004 Nov 6;4(1):9. doi: 10.1186/1472-6874-4-9. PMID: 15530170; PMCID: PMC534113.

2) ibid.

3) Zaira Donarelli, Gianluca Lo Coco, Salvatore Gullo, Angelo Marino, Andrea Volpes, Adolfo Allegra, Are attachment dimensions associated with infertility-related stress in couples undergoing their first IVF treatment? A study on the individual and cross-partner effect, Human Reproduction, Volume 27, Issue 11, November 2012, Pages 3215–3225, https://doi.org/10.1093/humrep/des307.

4) Patricia K. Kerig and Ava R. Alexander, "Models of Psychopathology," in Elsevier eBooks, 2023, https://doi.org/10.1016/b978-0-323-96023-6.00040-3.

5) Wikipedia contributors. "Psychological Pain." Wikipedia, April 12, 2024. https://en.wikipedia.org/wiki/Psychological_pain.

6) Kendra Cherry MSEd, "What Is the Fight-or-Flight Response?," Verywell Mind, November 7, 2022, https://www.verywellmind.com/what-is-the-fight-or-flight-response-2795194.

7) Martin Taylor, "What Does Fight, Flight, Freeze, Fawn Mean?," WebMD, April 28, 2022, https://www.webmd.com/mental-health/what-does-fight-flight-freeze-fawn-mean.

8) Melissa Kirk, "Why Do We Ruminate?: The functions rumination serves," Psychology Today, December 1, 2010, https://www.psychologytoday.com/us/blog/test-case/201012/why-do-we-ruminate

9) Sen, "Overcoming the Pain of Emotional Hurt | Calm Down Mind," May 30, 2011, https://www.calmdownmind.com/the-pain-of-emotional-hurt/.

10) Joann P. Galst Ph.D., "The Flip Side of Fertility Stress: Good news, finally," Psychology Today, August 26, 2017, https://www.psychologytoday.com/us/blog/fertility-factor/201708/ the-flip-side-fertility-stress.

11) Sevenmindsets. "Research & Results - 7 Mindsets." 7 Mindsets, May 2, 2024. https://7mindsets.com/research-results/.

12) Pao Chang, "The Power of Free Will and How to Use It to Change Your Fate," The Mind Unleashed (blog), March 31, 2015, https://themindunleashed.com/2015/03/the-power-of-free-will-and-how-to-use- it-to-change-your-fate.html.

13) "How to Fix a Broken Heart - Guy Winch," Guy Winch, March 10, 2021, https://www.guywinch.com/books/how-to-fix-a-broken-heart/.

14) Guy Winch Ph.D., "3 Surprising Ways Heartbreak Impacts Your Brain: When your heart gets broken, your brain does too.,"

Psychology Today, January 7, 2018, https://www.psychologytoday.com/us/blog/ the-squeaky-wheel/ 201801/3-surprising-ways-heartbreak-impacts-your-brain.

15) Wikipedia contributors, "Psychological Pain," Wikipedia, April 30, 2024, https://en.wikipedia.org/wiki/Psychological_pain.

Milton Keynes UK
Ingram Content Group UK Ltd.
UKHW041305181024
2256UKWH00002B/2